Doctors Who Cure Cancer: Anticancer Biography and New Way of Life to Treat the Emperor of All Maladies

Artour Rakhimov

Dr. Artour Rakhimov

Copyright ©2013 Artour Rakhimov.

All rights reserved.

This book is copyrighted. It is prohibited to copy, lend, adapt, electronically transmit, or transmit by any other means or methods without prior written approval from the author. However, the book may be borrowed by family members.

Disclaimer

The content provided herein is for information purposes only and not intended to diagnose, treat, cure or prevent cystic fibrosis or any other chronic disease. Always consult your doctor or health care provider before making any medical decisions). The information herein is the sole opinion of Dr. Artour Rakhimov and does not constitute medical advice. These statements have not been evaluated by Ontario Ministry of Health. Although every effort has been made to ensure the accuracy of the information herein, Dr. Artour Rakhimov accepts no responsibility or liability and makes no claims, promises, or guarantees about the accuracy, completeness, or adequacy of the information provided herein and expressly disclaims any liability for errors and omissions herein.

Table of Contents

Doctors Who Cure Cancer: Anticancer Biography and New Way of Life to Treat the Emperor of All Maladies

INTRODUCTION	5
1. BODY OXYGEN: THE KEY HEALTH FACTOR	7
1.1 Low body O2: the crucial factor in development of cancer	*8*
1.2 Acidic cellular pH or low body O2: what causes what?	*15*
1.3 Chronic inflammation and cancer	*19*
1.4 Inflammatory disorders are also based on low O2	*26*
1.5 Cell hypoxia causes oxidative stress and generation of free radicals	*30*
2. BREATHING NORMS VS. BREATHING IN PEOPLE WITH CANCER	35
2.1 Physiological norms for breathing at rest	*35*
2.2 Other parameters of normal breathing	*38*
2.3 Dr. Buteyko norms for breathing	*39*
2.4 Breathing parameters in people with cancer	*40*
3. EFFECTS OF OVERBREATHING (HYPERVENTILATION)	46
3.1 Vasoconstriction and reduced blood flow are caused by low CO2 in the arterial blood	*47*
3.2 Low CO2 results in the suppressed Bohr effect	*58*
3.3 Less oxygen for cells	*64*
3.4 Other effects of low arterial CO2	*67*
3.5 Are there any benefits from hyperventilation?	*70*
4. WHY CANCER IS COMMON NOW?	72
4.1 Breathing in ordinary people	*72*
4.2 Minute ventilation in healthy people	*81*
5. COMMON CO2 USES FOR CANCER TREATMENT	85
6. UKRAINIAN CLINICAL TRIAL: EFFECTS OF BREATHING NORMALIZATION ON METASTATIC BREAST CANCER	91
6.1 Metastatic cancer is deadly	*91*
6.2 Background and introduction	*94*
6.3 Subjects and methods of the trial	*96*
6.4 Results and discussion	*98*
6.5 The Buteyko method: chief self-oxygenation therapy	*101*
7. OTHER SELF-OXYGENATION THERAPIES	105
7.1 Frolov breathing device	*105*

7.2 How Does the Frolov Breathing Device Work? *109*
7.3 Amazing DIY breathing device *113*
7.4 Can yoga be used for self-oxygenation? *116*
7.5 Earthing: free electrons increase body O2 and fight tumors *120*
8. Conclusions 122
About the author: Dr. Artour Rakhimov 125

Introduction

This book does not claim that all metastatic cancers can be reversed. However, the initial stages of metastasis or spread of malignant cells to neighboring lymph nodes can be successfully addressed with therapies that increase body oxygenation naturally 24 hours a day, everyday. Russian and Ukrainian medical doctors applied their methods on hundreds of people with cancer and even had a published clinical trial on women with metastatic breast cancer. This trial was not an application of totally new techniques and methods for people with metastasis. Their protocol involved the application of additional therapies together with standard medical treatments such as surgery and radiation or chemotherapy. This trial clearly demonstrated the power of natural self-oxygenation methods, as well as the presence of dangerously low oxygen content in the participants of this trial before they applied those powerful self-oxygenation techniques. Cancer cannot exist in people with normal body O2 (oxygen) content.

The average oxygen concentration in cells of the body and within tumors is a known key factor that predicts appearance and aggressiveness of tumors. It is also a factor that in the survival of patients who are in the last stages of cancer. There are hundreds of recent medical studies that repeatedly claim that tissue hypoxia or low oxygenation of body cells plays the leading role in the development of cancer. These researchers and doctors do their research on a cellular level using very sophisticated techniques and methods to measure the effects of oxygen deprivation on malignant cells. They openly claim that they are clueless about the causes of tissue hypoxia which is found in each and each person with cancer.

However, the cause of the tissue hypoxia in people with cancer is their abnormal breathing. This has been discovered so far in each tested individual. What should happen if some physiological parameter is about 2 or more times away from the physiological standard? Imagine if one's heart rate were to beat twice as fast as normal or one's blood pressure were to increase to twice its normal range. Shouldn't it be a concern for people in the medical community and people who are involved in health care and treatment of diseases?. Wouldn't it be smart to address such deviations?

Oxygen does not appear in cells by itself or due to diffusion. The human respiratory system delivers oxygen to the lungs, then to blood and finally to tissues of the human body. If any part of the transportation system becomes slightly ineffective (for example, bringing only 1% less oxygen per minute), then after a certain time, the whole body starts to suffer from tissue hypoxia.
Cell hypoxia immediately generates a cascade of abnormal effects. Cell hypoxia causes cells to go into anaerobic respiration. Anaerobic respiration in cells elevates levels of lactic acid in blood, which then causes increased production of free radicals, promotes existing chronic inflammation, and leads to suppression of the immune system.

1. Body oxygen: the key health factor

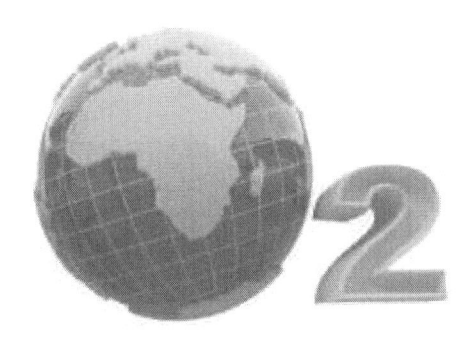

"All chronic pain, suffering and diseases are caused from a lack of oxygen at the cell level"
Guyton AC, The Textbook of Medical Physiology*, Fifth Edition

* World's most widely used medical textbook of any kind
* World's best-selling physiology book

Professor Guyton was the Dean of the University of Mississippi Medical School. This Guyton's quote suggests that chronic diseases require low body oxygenation. One cannot have normal body O2 concentrations and any chronic degenerative health problem. Let us consider the role of tissue hypoxia in case of cancer.

1.1 Low body O2: the crucial factor in development of cancer

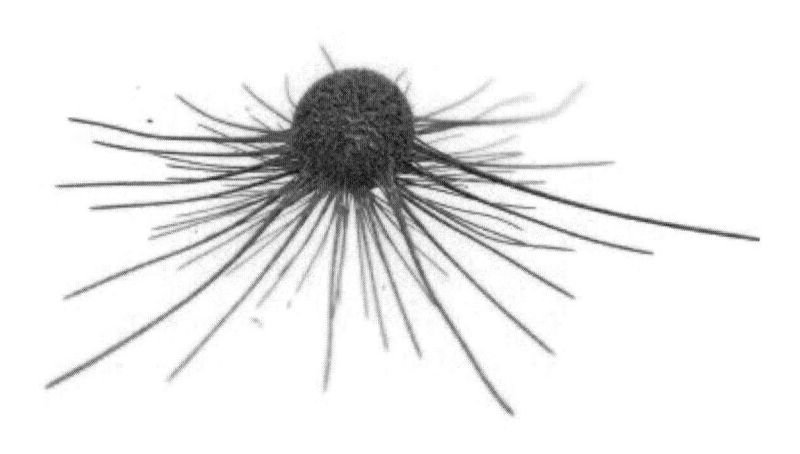

Nobel Laureate, Dr. Otto Warburg, in his Nobel Prize speech "The Prime Cause and Prevention of Cancer" (1966) stated, *"The prime cause of cancer is the replacement of the respiration of oxygen (oxidation of sugar) in normal body cells by fermentation of sugar... In every case, during the cancer development, the oxygen respiration always falls"*. Dr. Otto Warburg investigated the metabolism of tumors and the types of respiration of cells, particularly malignant cells. In 1931 he was awarded the Nobel Prize in Physiology and Medicine for his discovery of the *"nature and mode of action of the respiratory enzyme"*.

While Dr. Warburg only started the new era in molecular effects or micro causes of cancer (what is going on a cell level), there are numerous modern studies related to cellular causes of cancer. Many practitioners of alternative therapies suggest that cancer tumors appear and grow due to a pH which is too acidic within the cells of the human body. This acidic environment, as they assert, is created due to environmental influences where an abnormal diet with too much animal proteins and too little vegetables and grains plays the crucial role. While this idea of acidic dietary influences has some rational foundation, the real negative effects of excessive protein consumption are very different. We are going to explore this acidic pH idea and effects of diets in more detail later in this book. At the moment, let us focus on recent studies that explain the origins and cause of cancer.

First groups of cancer cells can appear only at low body O2

Why do first cancer cells appear? A group of microbiologists from the University of California in San Diego had the following title for their article: "*The hypoxia inducible factor-1 gene is required for embryogenesis and solid tumor formation*" (Ryan et al, 1998). As we can see from this title, tumors do not appear out of nowhere. They require low body oxygenation that is expressed in the hypoxia-inducible factor-1 that is the marker of low body oxygenation and a necessary factor for any first cancer cells to multiply and form a malignant tumor.

Cancer cells enjoy tissue hypoxia

Under normal conditions, even a group of hypoxic cells will die or will be easily destroyed by the immune system. What about cells in malignant tumors? Researchers from the Gray Laboratory Cancer Research Trust located in

Mount Vernon Hospital, Northwood, Middlesex, the UK concluded, *"Cells undergo a variety of biological responses when placed in hypoxic conditions, including activation of signaling pathways that regulate proliferation, angiogenesis and death. Cancer cells have adapted these pathways, allowing tumors to survive and even grow under hypoxic conditions..."* (Chaplin et al, 1986). These scientists say that cancer tumors like tissue hypoxia.

Here is another quote from a study done in the Yale University School of Medicine (USA). Dr Rockwell studied malignant changes on the cellular level and wrote, *"The physiological effects of hypoxia and the associated micro environmental inadequacies increase mutation rates, select for cells deficient in normal pathways of programmed cell death, and contribute to the development of an increasingly invasive, metastatic phenotype"* (Rockwell, 1997). The title of his publication is "*Oxygen delivery: implications for the biology and therapy of solid tumors*".

Low O2 is the crucial factor in cancer metastasis

When the solid tumor is large enough, and while body oxygenation becomes critically low, malignant cells start to invade neighboring lymph nodes and later other organs and tissues. This process is called metastasis.
Dozens of medical and physiological studies confirmed that low O2 concentrations in tumors and body cells control spread of malignant cells to other organs and tissues. Here is the title of one study that claims, "*Tumor oxygenation predicts for the likelihood of distant*

metastases in human soft tissue sarcoma" (Brizel et al, 1996).

German researchers from the the University of Leipzig and University of Rostock concluded, "*...Therefore, tissue hypoxia has been regarded as a central factor for tumor aggressiveness and metastasis*" (Kunz & Ibrahim, 2003). Canadian doctors from the Ontario Cancer Institute at the Princess Margaret Hospital (University of Toronto) even measured the effects of low body O2 values in chances of tumors to metastasize. These doctors found, "*In our studies of carcinoma of the cervix, nodal metastases were 1.5 times more likely at diagnosis in patients with more hypoxic tumours relative to those with less hypoxic tumours...*" (Hill et al, 2001)

Hypoxia and chances of survival

"*Clinical evidence shows that tumor hypoxia is an independent prognostic indicator of poor patient outcome. Hypoxic tumors have altered physiologic processes, including increased regions of angiogenesis, increased local invasion, increased distant metastasis and altered apoptotic programs*" (Denko et al, 2003).

Low O2 is a key parameter in treatment resistance

There are many therapies used by modern oncologists to treat cancers. Apart from radical treatment methods (or different forms of surgeries), there are other methods that include common conservative methods that include radiation therapy and chemotherapy. Obviously, medical professionals are trying to improve efficiency of these methods and find out causes of their low success rates.

Low cell O2 is one of the main factors that reduce success rates for chemotherapy and radiation therapy.
American scientists from Harvard Medical School noted "... *Hypoxia may thus produce both treatment resistance and a growth advantage*" (Schmaltz et al, 1998).
In their article published in Cancer Letters, Dr. Evans and Dr. Koch observed, "*Low tissue oxygen concentration has been shown to be important in the response of human tumors to radiation therapy, chemotherapy and other treatment modalities. Hypoxia is also known to be a prognostic indicator, as hypoxic human tumors are more biologically aggressive and are more likely to recur locally and metastasize*" (Evans & Koch, 2003).

Low O2 is the central factor in cancer dynamics

Growth of tumors and progression of any cancer is a dynamic process with changes that can take place within 5-10 minutes in both directions. We are going to provide practical examples related to this dynamic nature of cancer later. At the present moment, let us review relevant conclusions from recent medical and oncological research. German biologists from the Edinger Institute at the Johann Wolfgang Goethe University in Frankfurt directly claim, "*Thus mounting evidence suggests that the HIF [hypoxia-inducible factor] system plays a decisive role in tumor physiology and progression*" in their study "*A role for hypoxia and hypoxia-inducible transcription factors in tumor physiology*" (Acker & Plate, 2002).
French oncologists from the Institute of Signaling, Developmental Biology and Cancer Research at the University of Nice also reviewed the role of cell hypoxia in cancer dynamics. They wrote, "*Hypoxia is a common*

characteristic of the microenvironment of solid tumors and, through activation of the hypoxia-inducible factor, is at the center of the growth dynamics of tumor cells" (Dayan et al, 2008).

There is so much professional evidence about the fast growth of tumors when the condition of hypoxia is present that a large group of Californian researchers recently wrote a paper "*Hypoxia - inducible factor-1 is a positive factor in solid tumor growth*" (Ryan et al, 2000).
Echoing their paper, a British oncologist Dr. Harris from the Weatherhill Institute of Molecular Medicine (Oxford) went further with the manuscript "*Hypoxia - a key regulatory factor in tumor growth*" (Harris, 2002).

Conclusions

As we see from all these quoted studies, all stages of cancer from its birth and up to its death (and/or death of the owner) are tightly linked to O2 content in tumors and body cells. Note that I put these phrases together since body oxygenation and tumor oxygenation correlate with each other. When tumors grow, its low oxygenation exist on the background of whole body hypoxia that is an equal driving force for cancer development. If body oxygenation improves, due to some smart things that we can do, the tumor O2 content may not remain unaffected. Indeed, as we reviewed above, appearance of very first groups of cancer cells requires hypoxia that exist in normal (not malignant yet) cells.

References

Acker T, Plate KH *A role for hypoxia and hypoxia-inducible transcription factors in tumor physiology,* J Mol Med (Berlin). 2002 Sep;80(9):562-75.
Brizel DM, Scully SP, Harrelson JM, Layfield LJ, Bean JM, Prosnitz LR, Dewhirst MW, *Tumor oxygenation predicts for the likelihood of distant metastases in human soft tissue sarcoma,* Cancer Research 1996, 56: p. 941-943.
Dayan F, Mazure NM, Brahimi-Horn MC, Pouysségur J, *A dialogue between the hypoxia-inducible factor and the tumor microenvironment,* Cancer Microenviron. 2008 Dec;1(1):53-68.
Denko NC, Fontana LA, Hudson KM, Sutphin PD, Raychaudhuri S, Altman R, Giaccia AJ, *Investigating hypoxic tumor physiology through gene expression patterns,* Oncogene 2003 September 1; 22(37): p. 5907-5914.
Evans SM & Koch CJ, *Prognostic significance of tumor oxygenation in humans,* Cancer Letters 2003 May 30; 195(1): p. 1-16.
Harris AL, *Hypoxia: a key regulatory factor in tumor growth,* National Review in Cancer 2002 January; 2(1): p. 38-47.
Hill RP, De Jaeger K, Jang A, Cairns R, *pH, hypoxia and metastasis,* Novartis Found Symp. 2001;240:154-65; discussion 165-8.
Kunz M & Ibrahim SM, *Molecular responses to hypoxia in tumor cells,* Molecular Cancer 2003; 2: p. 23-31.
Rockwell S, *Oxygen delivery: implications for the biology and therapy of solid tumors,* Oncology Research 1997; 9(6-7): p. 383-390.

Ryan H, Lo J, Johnson RS, *The hypoxia inducible factor-1 gene is required for embryogenesis and solid tumor formation*, EMBO Journal 1998, 17: p. 3005-3015.
Ryan HE, Poloni M, McNulty W, Elson D, Gassmann M, Arbeit JM, Johnson RS, *Hypoxia-inducible factor-1 is a positive factor in solid tumor growth*, Cancer Res, August 1, 2000; 60(15): p. 4010 - 4015.*Hypoxia-inducible factor-1 is a positive factor in solid tumor growth*
Schmaltz C, Hardenbergh PH, Wells A, Fisher DE, *Regulation of proliferation-survival decisions during tumor cell hypoxia*, Molecular and Cellular Biology 1998 May, 18(5): p. 2845-2854.
Warburg O, *The Prime Cause and Prevention of Cancer*, Revised lecture at the meeting of the Nobel-Laureates on June 30, 1966.

1.2 Acidic cellular pH or low body O2: what causes what?

As it was mentioned above, many proponents of alternative therapies believe that cellular pH is the main factor that causes cancer tumors. Indeed, there are numerous studies that support the concept that tumor acidity is a significant factor that can prevent the success of conservative cancer treatment methods such as chemotherapy and radiation. Therefore, there are numerous websites and books which promote this idea and even offer treatment protocols to fight cancers. In this section of the book, we are going to review scientific evidence related to this topic: What is the primary factor in cancer growth: is it tissue hypoxia or acidic cellular pH? This question of cancer origins was analyzed in numerous published studies on cancer. A group of American doctors from the Department of Medicine and the Cancer Center at the University of California in La Jolla in their conclusions wrote, "*These results indicate that hypoxia and its accompanying low pH enrich for MMR-deficient cells and that loss of MMR renders human colon carcinoma cells hypersensitive to the ability of hypoxia to induce microsatellite instability and generate highly drug-resistant clones in the surviving population*" (Kondo et al, 2001).

A team of scientists from the Cancer Research Institute at the University of Nice in France devoted their publication to the following topic, "*A dialogue between the hypoxia-inducible factor and the tumor microenvironment*" (Dayan et al, 2008). In their abstract, they wrote, "*Hypoxia is a common characteristic of the microenvironment of solid tumors and, through activation of the hypoxia-inducible factor, is at the center of the growth dynamics of tumor cells. Not only does the microenvironment impact on the hypoxia-inducible factor but this factor impacts on microenvironmental features, such as pH, nutrient availability, metabolism and the extracellular matrix.*" We can see here that the answer is simple.

Low cellular O2 causes abnormal pH changes.

Californian researcher Dr. Payne from the Steenblock Research Institute suggested the exact mechanism how tissue hypoxia causes low intracellular pH. "*Chemo- and radio-resistant cancer cells within solid tumors undermine the effectiveness of these approaches to achieving oncolysis. These resistant cells and clusters of cells typically thrive at low oxygen tensions and are reliant on anaerobic metabolic pathways that churn out lactate. This hypoxic state is one that can be exploited and in this paper a novel method is advanced involving tumor cell infiltration by bifidobacterium species which should bring about prodigious lactate synthesis; concomitant blocking of its enzymatic degradation by urea as well as export (from the cell) by use of quercetin; depletion of ATP using exogenous thyroid; and compromised oxidative catabolism of free fatty acids and amino acids via oral intake of l-hydroxycitrate, melatonin and nontoxic NDGA. This "anaerobic pathway cocktail", it is hypothesized, will bring about a profound reduction in intracellular pH and a compromised state of cellular energetics sufficient to effect oncolysis"* (Payne, 2007).

Italian scientists from Rome were also interested, according to the title of their article in *"Tumor acidity, chemoresistance and proton pump inhibitors"*. They wrote, *"An important determinant of tumor acidity is the anaerobic metabolism that allows selection of cells able to survive in an hypoxic-anoxic environment with the generation of lactate"* (De Milito & Fais, 2005). As we see, they also suggest that anaerobic respiration of cells causes acidity in tumors.

British Oxford researchers from the Imperial Cancer Research Fund at the University of Oxford (Institute of Molecular Medicine) pinpointed the key trigger of pathological events leading to advance of cancers. *"Hypoxia, a common consequence of solid tumor growth in breast cancer and other cancers, serves to propagate a cascade of molecular pathways which include angiogenesis, glycolysis, and alterations in microenvironmental pH..."* (Goonewardene et al, 2002).

A study by German oncologists published in the Journal of Molecular Medicine confirmed the same conclusion about the primary driving force of cancers. The researchers wrote, "*The HIF system induces adaptive responses including angiogenesis, glycolysis, and pH regulation which confer increased resistance towards the hostile tumor microenvironment*" (Acker & Plate, 2002).
To my knowledge, there are no studies that suggest or confirm the leading role of cellular pH in creation of cell hypoxia or in cancer dynamics. There are indeed numerous studies claiming that low pH or acidic environment of tumors is a very potent negative factor that makes acidic tumors very resistant to all types of conservative treatments.

Many proponents of alternative therapies promote an idea that cancer is caused by a poor diet with too many acidic foods that makes cells acidic and leads to growth of tumors. This is the influence of acidic diets which are usually based on animal proteins and junk foods. However, these effects are not due to this nearly mechanical hypothetical relationship: you eat more amino acids and less foods with minerals, therefore you get acidic body cells. The negative mechanism due to excessive dietary proteins, especially animal proteins in comparison with vegetables, fruits and other foods that have less amino acids but more minerals and other nutrients, is very different. There is some rationality in having vegetarian diets provided that all required nutrients are provided. Medical research showed that diets based on animal proteins make breathing heavier in comparison with vegetarian diets. Heavy breathing, as we are going to learn later, reduces body and tumor oxygenation.

References

Acker T, Plate KH *A role for hypoxia and hypoxia-inducible transcription factors in tumor physiology,* J Mol Med (Berlin). 2002 Sep;80(9):562-75.

Dayan F, Mazure NM, Brahimi-Horn MC, Pouysségur J, *A dialogue between the hypoxia-inducible factor and the tumor microenvironment,* Cancer Microenviron. 2008 Dec;1(1):53-68.

De Milito A, Fais S, *Tumor acidity, chemoresistance and proton pump inhibitors,* Future Oncol. 2005 Dec;1(6):779-86.

Goonewardene TI, Sowter HM, Harris AL, *Hypoxia-induced pathways in breast cancer,* Microsc Res Tech. 2002 Oct 1;59(1):41-8.
Payne AG, *Exploiting hypoxia in solid tumors to achieve oncolysis,* Med Hypotheses. 2007;68(4):828-31.

1.3 Chronic inflammation and cancer

When we consider only appearance of inflamed tissues, we can immediately suspect that these swollen inflamed cells have some features that make them similar to malignant cells. Rudolph Carl Virchow (1821 – 1902) was a famous German doctor, anthropologist, pathologist, and biologist was probably the first doctor who in 1863 suggested the link between chronic inflammation and cancer. He demonstrated leucocytes in neoplastic tissue. Dr. Virchow is often referred to as "the father of modern pathology" and considered one of the founders of social medicine. Recent modern oncological studies have also confirmed the link using a more detailed description of events leading to chronic inflammation and appearance of malignant tumors. There are several common key chemicals that are parts of chronic inflammatory and developing malignant processes. Furthermore, many researchers found that having inflammatory health problems increase chances of cancer. Many oncologists suggested that chronic inflammation is even one the key factors causing cancer. For example, doctors from the The Sidney Kimmel Comprehensive Cancer Center in Baltimore, MD wrote, "*Chronic inflammation is now known to contribute to several forms of human cancer, with an estimated 20% of adult cancers attributable to chronic inflammatory conditions caused by infectious agents, chronic non-infectious inflammatory diseases and/or other environmental factors. Indeed, chronic inflammation is now regarded as an 'enabling characteristic' of human cancer*" (Sfanos & De Marzo, 2012).

Australian scientists from Melbourne (Peter MacCallum Cancer Centre and Department of Oncology at the University of Melbourne) also observed, "*Chronic inflammation is a risk factor for tumor development*" (Chow et al, 2012).

Dr. Morrison provided several common chemicals that explain why chronic inflammation promotes growth of cancers, "*... chronic inflammation and associated reactive free radical overload and some types of bacterial, viral, and parasite infections that cause inflammation were* *recognized as important risk factors for cancer development and account for one in four of all human cancers worldwide. Even viruses that do not directly cause inflammation can cause cancer when they act in conjunction with proinflammatory cofactors or when they initiate or promote cancer via the same signaling pathways utilized in inflammation. Whatever its origin, inflammation in the tumor microenvironment has many cancer-promoting effects and aids in the proliferation and survival of malignant cells and promotes angiogenesis and metastasis. Mediators of inflammation such as cytokines, free radicals, prostaglandins, and growth factors can induce DNA damage in tumor suppressor genes and post-translational modifications of proteins involved in essential cellular processes including apoptosis, DNA repair, and cell cycle checkpoints that can lead to initiation and progression of cancer"* (Morrison, 2012).

Korean oncologists from the Cancer Research Institute at the Seoul National University devoted their review, according to the title of their recent article to *"Inflammation: gearing the journey to cancer"* (Kundu & Surh, 2008). In their summary, they wrote, "*Many of proinflammatory mediators, especially cytokines, chemokines and prostaglandins, turn on the angiogenic switches mainly controlled by vascular endothelial growth factor, thereby inducing inflammatory angiogenesis and tumor cell-stroma communication. This will end up with tumor angiogenesis, metastasis and invasion. Moreover, cellular microRNAs are emerging as a potential link between inflammation and cancer*".

Another title of the research paper written by researchers from the Department of Molecular and Biomedical Pharmacology at University of Kentucky School of Medicine in Lexington also suggests the same story *"Inflammation: a driving force speeds cancer metastasis"* (Wu & Zhou, 2009).

Drs. Hofseth and Wargovich from the Department of Basic Pharmaceutical Sciences at the South Carolina College of Pharmacy also specified key chemicals that participate in promotion of chronic inflammation and development of cancer. *"At the molecular level, free radicals and aldehydes, produced during chronic inflammation, can induce deleterious gene mutation and posttranslational modifications of key cancer-related proteins. Other products of inflammation, including cytokines, growth factors, and transcription factors such as nuclear factor kappaB, control the expression of cancer genes (e.g., suppressor genes and oncogenes) and key inflammatory enzymes such as inducible nitric oxide synthase and cyclooxygenase-2. These enzymes in turn directly influence reactive oxygen species and eicosanoid levels. The procancerous outcome of chronic inflammation is increased DNA damage, increased DNA synthesis, cellular proliferation, disruption of DNA repair pathways and cellular milieu, inhibition of apoptosis, and promotion of angiogenesis and invasion. Chronic inflammation is also associated with immunosuppression, which is a risk factor for cancer"* (Hofseth & Wargovich, 2007)

There are so many similarities between chronic inflammation and cancer, that many teams of scientists are even trying the same medical drugs and natural extracts or substances to combat both these conditions. This relates to application of:

- andrographolide and its analogues (Lim et al, 2012)

- curcumin (Schaffer et al, 2011)

- folic acid that is also known as vitamin B9 (Yang et al, 2012),

- tocotrienols, the potent isoforms of vitamin E (Nesaretnam & Meganathan, 2011)

- thymoquinone, an active ingredient isolated from Nigella sativa (Woo et al, 2012)

- unstable naturally derived hepoxilins, metabolites of arachidonic acid (Pace-Asciak, 2011)

- group of autacoid mediators that are the products of arachidonic acid metabolism include: the prostaglandins, leukotrienes, lipoxins and cytochrome P450 (CYP) derived bioactive products, which are all collectively referred to as eicosanoids (Greene et al, 2011)

- resveratrol (trans-3,4',5-trihydroxystilbene), a natural polyphenol with antioxidant, anti-inflammatory, and anticancer properties (Tili & Michaille, 2011)
and some other substances.

While application of these products may have certain beneficial chemical reactions, without removal of the key cause of low body O2 levels, their overall efficiency will be very low. Note that there are often true stories of people testifying about their magic recovery following use of some special protocols. However, when other people with cancer apply to the same substances using the same dosages, very few of them are able to achieve the same results. The effects of various positive substances and functional foods depends on body oxygen levels that can be easily measured using the body oxygen test described below.

References

Chow MT, Möller A, Smyth MJ, *Inflammation and immune surveillance in cancer,* Semin Cancer Biol. 2012 Feb;22(1):23-32.

Greene ER, Huang S, Serhan CN, Panigrahy D, *Regulation of inflammation in cancer by eicosanoids,* Prostaglandins Other Lipid Mediat. 2011 Nov;96(1-4):27-36.

Hofseth LJ, Wargovich MJ, *Inflammation, cancer, and targets of ginseng,* J Nutr. 2007 Jan;137(1 Suppl):183S-185S.

Kundu JK, Surh YJ, *Inflammation: gearing the journey to cancer,* Mutat Res. 2008 Jul-Aug;659(1-2):15-30.

Lim JC, Chan TK, Ng DS, Sagineedu SR, Stanslas J, Wong WF, *Andrographolide and its analogues: versatile bioactive molecules for combating inflammation and cancer,* Clin Exp Pharmacol Physiol. 2012 Mar;39(3):300-10.

Morrison WB, *Inflammation and cancer: a comparative view,* J Vet Intern Med. 2012 Jan-Feb;26(1):18-31.

Nesaretnam K, Meganathan P, *Tocotrienols: inflammation and cancer,* Ann N Y Acad Sci. 2011 Jul;1229:18-22.

Pace-Asciak CR, *Hepoxilins in cancer and inflammation-- use of hepoxilin antagonists,* Cancer Metastasis Rev. 2011 Dec;30(3-4):493-506.
Schaffer M, Schaffer PM, Zidan J, Bar Sela G, *Curcuma as a functional food in the control of cancer and inflammation,* Curr Opin Clin Nutr Metab Care. 2011 Nov;14(6):588-97.

Sfanos KS, De Marzo AM, *Prostate cancer and inflammation: the evidence.* Histopathology. 2012 Jan;60(1):199-215.

Tili E, Michaille JJ, *Resveratrol, MicroRNAs, Inflammation, and Cancer,* J Nucleic Acids. 2011;2011:102431.

Woo CC, Kumar AP, Sethi G, Tan KH, *Thymoquinone: potential cure for inflammatory disorders and cancer,*

Biochem Pharmacol. 2012 Feb 15;83(4):443-51.
Wu Y, Zhou BP, *Inflammation: a driving force speeds cancer metastasis,* Cell Cycle. 2009 Oct 15;8(20):3267-73.

Yang J, Vlashi E, Low P, *Folate-linked drugs for the treatment of cancer and inflammatory diseases,* Subcell Biochem. 2012;56:163-79.

1.4 Inflammatory disorders are also based on low O2

As numerous very recent studies claim, chronic inflammatory conditions, on a cell level, are also controlled by tissue hypoxia or low oxygen content in cells. Among the key driving forces of chronic inflammation are pro-inflammatory transcription factors, such as nuclear factor kappa B (NF-kappaB), activator protein (AP)-1 (Safronova & Morita, 2010; Ryan et al, 2009), and *hypoxia-inducible factor* 1 (Imtiyaz & Simon, 2010; Sumbayev & Nicholas, 2010), the same substance that is the key factor in cancer (see Part 1.1).

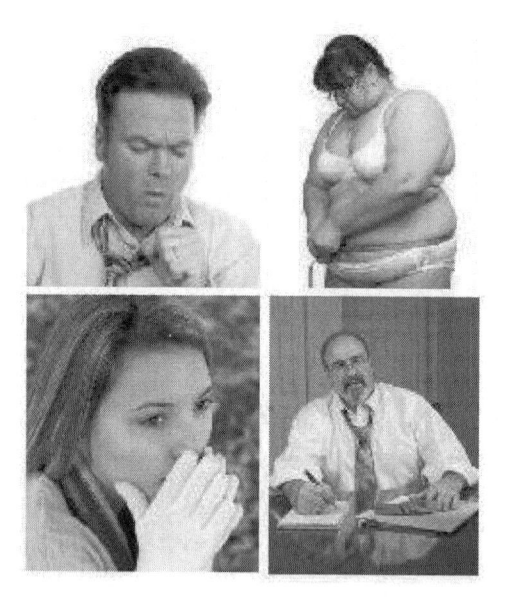

Both effects, chronic inflammation and low oxygen levels in cells, are common in people with many chronic diseases, such as:
- arthritic conditions
- Alzheimer's disease
- asthma

- autoimmune diseases
- acne
- allergic reactions
- atherosclerosis
- chronic prostatitis
- Crohn's disease
- COPD
- dermatitis
- hepatitis
- hypersensitivities and allergic reactions
- insulin resistance (diabetes)
- irritable bowel syndrome (IBS) of the intestinal tract
- inflammatory bowel diseases (IBD)
- lupus
- nephritis
- obesity
- cachexia
- gastrointestinal ischemia
- osteoarthritis
- pelvic inflammatory disease
- Parkinson's disease
- sarcoidosis
- sleep apnea
- transplant rejection
- and ulcerative colitis.

Symptoms of these chronic diseases include inflammation, possible fatigue due to exhausted cortisol reserves, likely pain, and other symptoms. Several other chronic diseases (including atherosclerosis, and ischemic heart disease) also have their origins in chronic inflammatory processes. The same is true for cancer as we discussed above. There are hundreds of research studies that either mentioned or proved the facts provided above. Some of these studies are listed below.

References

Arnaud C, Dematteis M, Pepin JL, Baguet JP, Lévy P, *Obstructive sleep apnea, immuno-inflammation, and atherosclerosis,* Semin Immunopathol. 2009 Jun;31(1):113-25.

Eltzschig HK, Rivera-Nieves J, Colgan SP, *Targeting the A2B adenosine receptor during gastrointestinal ischemia and inflammation,* Expert Opin Ther Targets. 2009 Nov;13(11):1267-77.

Frede S, Berchner-Pfannschmidt U, Fandrey J, *Regulation of hypoxia-inducible factors during inflammation,* Methods Enzymol. 2007;435:405-19.

Imtiyaz HZ, Simon MC, *Hypoxia-inducible factors as essential regulators of inflammation,* Curr Top Microbiol

Immunol. 2010;345:105-20.

Joussen AM, Fauser S, Krohne TU, Lemmen KD, Lang GE, Kirchhof B, *Diabetic retinopathy. Pathophysiology and therapy of hypoxia-induced inflammation* [Article in German], Ophthalmologe. 2003 May;100(5):363-70.

Oliver KM, Taylor CT, Cummins EP, *Hypoxia. Regulation of NFkappaB signalling during inflammation: the role of hydroxylases,* Arthritis Res Ther. 2009;11(1):215.

Ramalho R, Guimarães C, *The role of adipose tissue and macrophages in chronic inflammation associated with obesity: clinical implications* [Article in Portuguese], Acta Med Port. 2008 Sep-Oct;21(5):489-96. Epub 2009 Jan 16.

Ryan S, Taylor CT, McNicholas WT, *Systemic inflammation: a key factor in the pathogenesis of cardiovascular complications in obstructive sleep apnoea syndrome?* Thorax. 2009 Jul;64(7):631-6.

Safronova O, Morita I, *Transcriptome remodeling in hypoxic inflammation,* J Dent Res. 2010 May;89(5):430-44. Epub 2010 Mar 26.

Sumbayev VV, Nicholas SA, *Hypoxia-inducible factor 1 as one of the "signaling drivers" of Toll-like receptor-dependent and allergic inflammation,* Arch Immunol Ther Exp (Warsz). 2010 Aug;58(4):287-94. Epub 2010 May 26. Taylor CT, *Interdependent roles for hypoxia inducible factor and nuclear factor-kappaB in hypoxic inflammation,* J Physiol. 2008 Sep 1;586(Pt 17):4055-9.

Wouters EF, *Local and systemic inflammation in chronic obstructive pulmonary disease,* Proc Am Thorac Soc. 2005;2(1):26-33.

1.5 Cell hypoxia causes oxidative stress and generation of free radicals

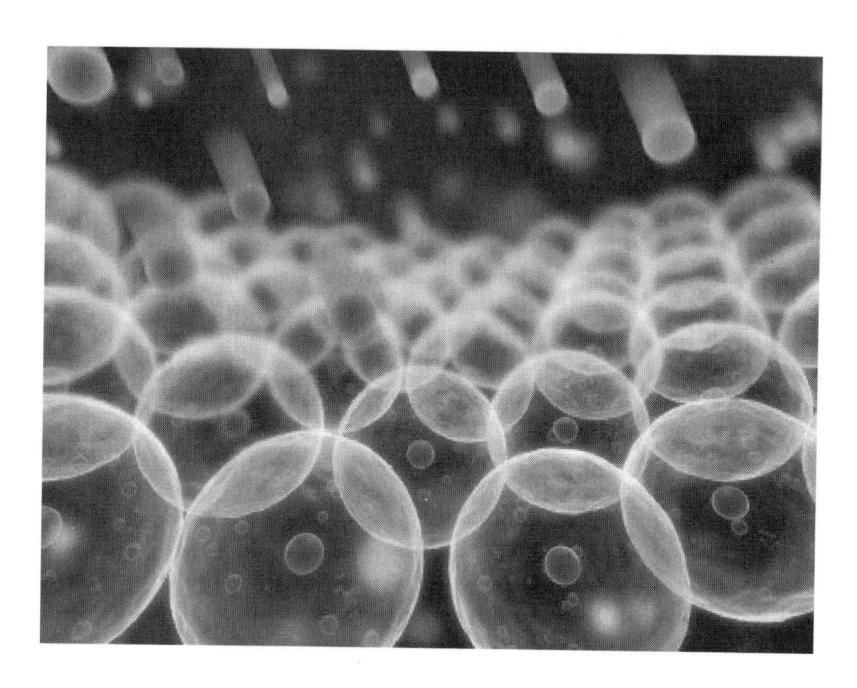

When oxygen supply is restricted, it is necessary for various bodily processes and reactions to take place in cells and organs, there are various protective but damaging mechanisms and solutions that maintain vital functions in various parts of the human body. These adaptations to cell hypoxia are different in various organs of the human body and, in addition, are specific in duration. These are the conclusions of the study titled *"Intermittent hypoxia has organ-specific effects on oxidative stress"* (Jun J, Savransky et al, 2008) conducted at the John Hopkins Asthma and Allergy Center, Division of Pulmonology and Critical Care Medicine in Baltimore, MD, USA.

Furthermore, hypoxia-induced chemicals can be generated in some areas and parts of the human body but cause problems for other organs, for example, the brain and heart.

However, there are common mechanisms related to effects of tissue hypoxia. You have probably heard about antioxidants and free radicals. Free radicals are also called "reactive oxygen species" (those powerful chemicals that can cause damage to hundreds or thousands of other cells due to their inherent destructive power). They create so called "oxygen stress". Maybe you even take supplements that contain such known and popular antioxidants as vitamin C, zinc, vitamin A, selenium and some others. However, it is very likely that you generate free radicals in your body cells due to your ineffective or abnormal breathing.

Why do researchers call it "oxygen stress"? Normal air has only about 20% of oxygen, while the main remaining part is neutral nitrogen that is an inert gas. Pure oxygen (or 100% oxygen), as any respirologist can tell you, is toxic due to its powerful abilities to react with tissues. The damage due to breathing pure oxygen and especially hyperbaric breathing starts in the lungs. Right oxygen is bound with red blood cells (or hemoglobin cells). It is released in tissues and safely transported to required cells and parts of the cell. Obviously, any attempts to consume oxygenated drinks, oxygenated bars, or even breathing hyperoxic air (more than 20% at normal pressure) can be life-saving for critically ill people, but always leads to worse health in a long run.

Let us now consider other well-proven effects of hypoxia related to generation of free radicals. Abnormally low oxygen delivery leads to anaerobic (i.e., without participation of oxygen) cellular respiration, generation of lactic acid and free radicals. There are hundreds of research studies that claim that generation of free radicals is a normal and known outcome of cell hypoxia. (Note that some studies simulated cell hypoxia by reducing oxygen content in the inspired air, but breathing abnormalities present in most people cause exactly the same effect: low body O2 content.) There are only some references that are provided below. Their titles clearly highlight the role of hypoxia in generation of free radicals.

References

Carvalho C, Santos MS, Baldeiras I, Oliveira CR, Seiça R, Moreira PI, *Chronic hypoxia potentiates age-related oxidative imbalance in brain vessels and synaptosomes,* Curr Neurovasc Res. 2010 Nov;7(4):288-300.

Dukhande VV, Sharma GC, Lai JC, Farahani R, *Chronic hypoxia-induced alterations of key enzymes of glucose oxidative metabolism in developing mouse liver are mTOR dependent,* Mol Cell Biochem. 2011 Nov;357(1-2):189-97.

Esteva S, Pedret R, Fort N, Torrella JR, Pagès T, Viscor G, *Oxidative stress status in rats after intermittent exposure to hypobaric hypoxia,* Wilderness Environ Med. 2010 Dec;21(4):325-31.

Favaro E, Ramachandran A, McCormick R, Gee H, Blancher C, Crosby M, Devlin C, Blick C, Buffa F, Li JL,

Vojnovic B, Pires das Neves R, Glazer P, Iborra F, Ivan M, Ragoussis J, Harris AL, *MicroRNA-210 regulates mitochondrial free radical response to hypoxia and Krebs cycle in cancer cells by targeting iron sulfur cluster protein ISCU,* PLoS One. 2010 Apr 26;5(4):e10345.

Giordano FJ, *Oxygen, oxidative stress, hypoxia, and heart failure,* J Clin Invest. 2005 Mar;115(3):500-8.

Himadri P, Kumari SS, Chitharanjan M, Dhananjay S, *Role of oxidative stress and inflammation in hypoxia-induced cerebral edema: a molecular approach,* High Alt Med Biol. 2010 Fall;11(3):231-44.

Jun J, Savransky V, Nanayakkara A, Bevans S, Li J, Smith PL, Polotsky VY, *Intermittent hypoxia has organ-specific effects on oxidative stress,* Am J Physiol Regul Integr Comp Physiol. 2008 Oct;295(4):R1274-81.

Martin R, Mozet C, Martin H, Welt K, Engel C, Fitzl G, *The effect of Ginkgo biloba extract (EGb 761) on parameters of oxidative stress in different regions of aging rat brains after acute hypoxia,* Aging Clin Exp Res. 2011 Aug;23(4):255-63.

Mustafa SA, Al-Subiai SN, Davies SJ, Jha AN, *Hypoxia-induced oxidative DNA damage links with higher level biological effects including specific growth rate in common carp, Cyprinus carpio L,* Ecotoxicology. 2011 Aug;20(6):1455-66.

Patterson AJ, Xiao D, Xiong F, Dixon B, Zhang L, *Hypoxia-derived oxidative stress mediates epigenetic repression of PKC{varepsilon} gene in foetal rat hearts.* Cardiovasc Res. 2012 Feb 1;93(2):302-10.

Pialoux V, Foster GE, Ahmed SB, Beaudin AE, Hanly PJ, Poulin MJ, *Losartan abolishes oxidative stress induced by intermittent hypoxia in humans,* J Physiol. 2011 Nov 15;589(Pt 22):5529-37.

Ramond A, Godin-Ribuot D, Ribuot C, Totoson P, Koritchneva I, Cachot S, Levy P, Joyeux-Faure M, *Oxidative stress mediates cardiac infarction aggravation induced by intermittent hypoxia,* Fundam Clin Pharmacol. 2011 Dec 7. doi: 10.1111/j.1472-8206.

Skoumalová A, Herget J, Wilhelm J, *Hypercapnia protects erythrocytes against free radical damage induced by hypoxia in exposed rats,* Cell Biochem Funct. 2008 Oct;26(7):801-7.

Xu J, Long YS, Gozal D, Epstein PN, *Beta-cell death and proliferation after intermittent hypoxia: role of oxidative stress,* Free Radic Biol Med. 2009 Mar 15;46(6):783-90.

2. Breathing norms vs. breathing in people with cancer

Each and every person with cancer has ineffective or abnormal breathing pattern that reduces their body oxygenation. We can make this conclusion from all studies that measured automatic breathing patterns in people with cancer, as well as from clinical experience of medical doctors and health practitioners who measured breathing in their patients and clients.
In order to investigate and understand what is wrong with breathing in people with cancers, let us start with an analysis of medical norms for breathing at rest, as well as typical respiratory parameters in healthy and ordinary people. Later, we are going to consider those studies that measured various breathing parameters in people with cancer.

2.1 Physiological norms for breathing at rest

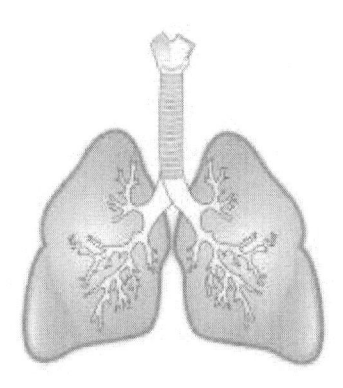

Normal breathing is strictly nasal (in and out), predominantly diaphragmatic (i.e., abdominal), very slow in frequency (see the numbers below) and imperceptible (no feelings or sensation about one's own breathing at rest; see the explanation below). The physiological norm for minute ventilation at rest is 6 liters of air for one minute for a 70 kg man, as numerous physiological textbooks indicate (e.g., Guyton, 1984; Ganong, 1995; and Straub, 1998). These medical textbooks also provide the following parameters for normal breathing:

- normal breathing frequency is 12 breaths per minute
- normal tidal volume (air volume breathed in during a single breath) is 500 ml
- normal inspiration is about 2 seconds
- normal exhalation is about 3 seconds.

To be more accurate, the normal inhalation is little bit shorter or about 1.5 seconds, while the exhalation is longer or nearly 3.5 seconds. The following graph represents the normal breathing pattern at rest or the dynamic of the air volume in the lungs as a function of time:

Amount of air in the lungs, ml

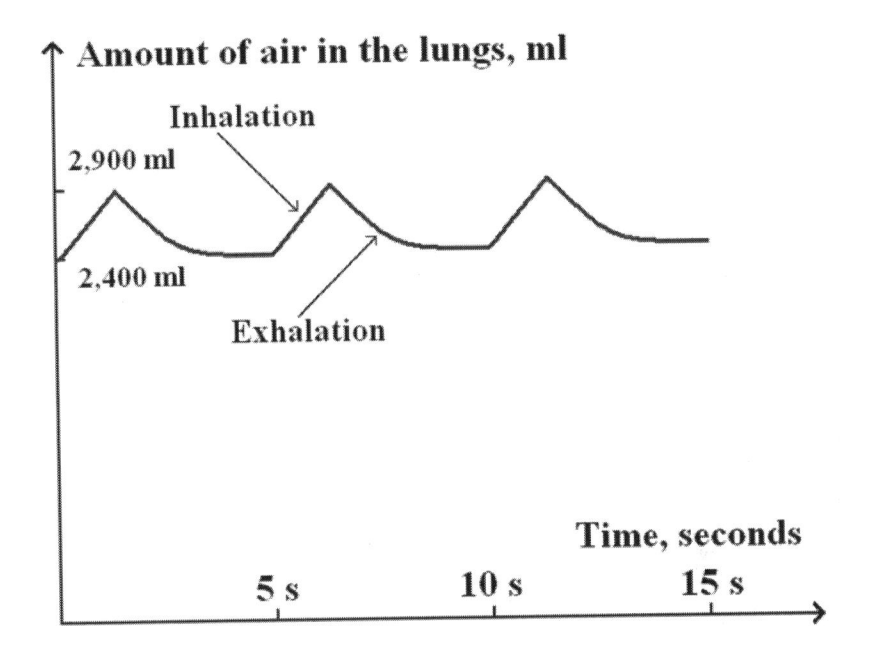

- 2,900 ml
- Inhalation
- 2,400 ml
- Exhalation

Time, seconds: 5 s, 10 s, 15 s

If a person with normal breathing is asked about what they feel or their breathing sensations, they will testify that they do not feel their breathing at all (unless their practice yoga breathing or some other breathing exercises). Why is this so? Normal tidal volume is only 500 ml or about 0.6 g of air, which is inhaled during one inspiration. Hence, normal breathing is slow in frequency and very small in amplitude.

References (Medical and physiological textbooks)

Ganong WF, *Review of medical physiology*, 15-th ed., 1995, Prentice Hall Int., London.

Guyton AC, *Physiology of the human body*, 6-th ed., 1984, Suanders College Publ., Philadelphia.

Straub NC, *Section V, The Respiratory System, in Physiology*, eds. RM Berne & MN Levy, 4-th edition, Mosby, St. Louis, 1998.
Summary of values useful in pulmonary physiology: man. Section: Respiration and Circulation, ed. by P.L. Altman & D.S. Dittmer, 1971, Bethesda, Maryland (Federation of American Societies for Experimental Biology).

2.2 Other parameters of normal breathing

"If a person breath-holds after a normal exhalation, it takes about 40 seconds before breathing commences" (McArdle et al, 2000). This 40 seconds indicate normal oxygenation of tissues. Note that the breath holding test is done after usual exhalation.

The current medical norm for CO_2 content in the alveoli of the lungs and the arterial blood is 40 mm Hg CO_2. This number was established during the first decade of the 20th century by famous British physiologists Charles G. Douglas and John S. Haldane from Oxford University.

Their results were published in 1909 article "*The regulation of normal breathing*" by the Journal of Physiology (Douglas & Haldane, 1909). This corresponds to about 5.3% (at sea level). You do not need to remember all these numbers. They are going to be used only to show that cancer patients never have these norms.

Let me note here that normal CO_2 in the arterial blood is absolutely necessary for normal transport of oxygen to cells. We are going to discuss the reasons later.

Normal breathing is regular, invisible (no chest or belly movements), mainly diaphragmatic, and inaudible (no panting, no wheezing, no sighing, no yawning, no sneezing, no coughing, no deep inhalations or exhalations).

According to numerous medical textbooks, this very small and slow normal diaphragmatic breathing leads to nearly ideal oxygenation of the arterial blood: about 98-99%. This conclusion is important for future since many people believe in a myth that deep breathing or breathing more air helps to increase blood oxygenation. In reality, one can breathe 3-5 times more than the morn, but blood oxygenation will not be improved to any essential degree. In fact, since chronic automatic overbreathing leads to chest breathing, while lower parts of the lungs get about 5-6 times more blood due to gravity, **overbreathing usually reduces blood oxygenation**.

References

Douglas CG, Haldane JS, *The regulation of normal breathing*, Journal of Physiology 1909; 38: p. 420–440.
McArdle W.D., Katch F.I., Katch V.L., *Essentials of exercise physiology* (2-nd edition); Lippincott, Williams and Wilkins, London 2000.

2.3 Dr. Buteyko norms for breathing

During the 1960's for nearly the whole decade, Soviet Dr. Konstantin Buteyko (born in Ukraine) was the manager of the respiratory laboratory in Novosibirsk (USSR). Based on his studies of thousands of healthy and sick people in this laboratory, he suggested different norms for breathing (e.g., Buteyko, 1991) that guarantee excellent health and absence of nearly all chronic degenerative diseases, cancer included. What are his medical norms? For example, his normal respiratory rate is only 8 breaths/min instead of 12. Here are his numbers for normal breathing:

- normal minute ventilation is 4 l/min;
- normal tidal volume (air volume breathed in during a single breath) is 500 ml;
- normal breathing rate or respiratory frequency is 8 breaths per minute;
- inspiration is about 1.5 seconds;
- exhalation is 2 seconds;
- automatic pause (or period of no breathing after exhalation) is 4 seconds;
- breath holding time (after usual exhalation and without any stress at the end of the test) is 60 seconds;
- CO_2 concentrations in the alveoli or arterial blood is 6.5% or about 46 mm Hg (at sea level).

As we are going to study later, such easy and slow automatic breathing at rest delivers more oxygen to tissues of the human body than the current official medical norm accepted all over the world.

2.4 Breathing parameters in people with cancer

All available medical literature clearly demonstrates that virtually all people with cancer have ineffective or abnormal breathing. In one study conducted by the Division of Respiratory and Critical Care Medicine at the Department of Medicine of the Queen's University in Kingston (Ontario, Canada), researchers measured minute ventilation in people with cancer (Travers et al, 2008). The scientists were actually interested in respiratory differences related to presence of dyspnea that is one of the symptoms in cancer patients. However, minute ventilation in participants of this study was the same regardless the presence of dyspnea. Both cancer groups (40 participants in total) had about 12±2 liters of air per minute at rest, while the medical norm for adults is about 6 liters per minute. All these cancer patients also had elevated breathing frequency of about 19-20 breaths/min instead of normal 12 breaths/min.

Obviously, when one breathes or ventilates much more than the physiological norm, it is called "hyperventilation". It would be logical to expect that their overbreathing caused low CO_2 levels in the airways and the arterial blood.

This Canadian study allows us to calculate the amount of air per one breath in people with cancer. Since the participants had about 12 liters per minute with nearly 20 breaths per minute, we can divide 12 by 20 and get 0.6 liters for one breath or 600 ml of air for their tidal volume. The normal value is 500 ml. Therefore, we see that this group of cancer patients were breathing deeply at rest. They breathing was faster and deeper than the medical norms.

Several other studies measured respiratory frequency at rest in patients with cancer who experienced dyspnea. All the results of these studies are summarized in this graph.

Dr. Artour Rakhimov

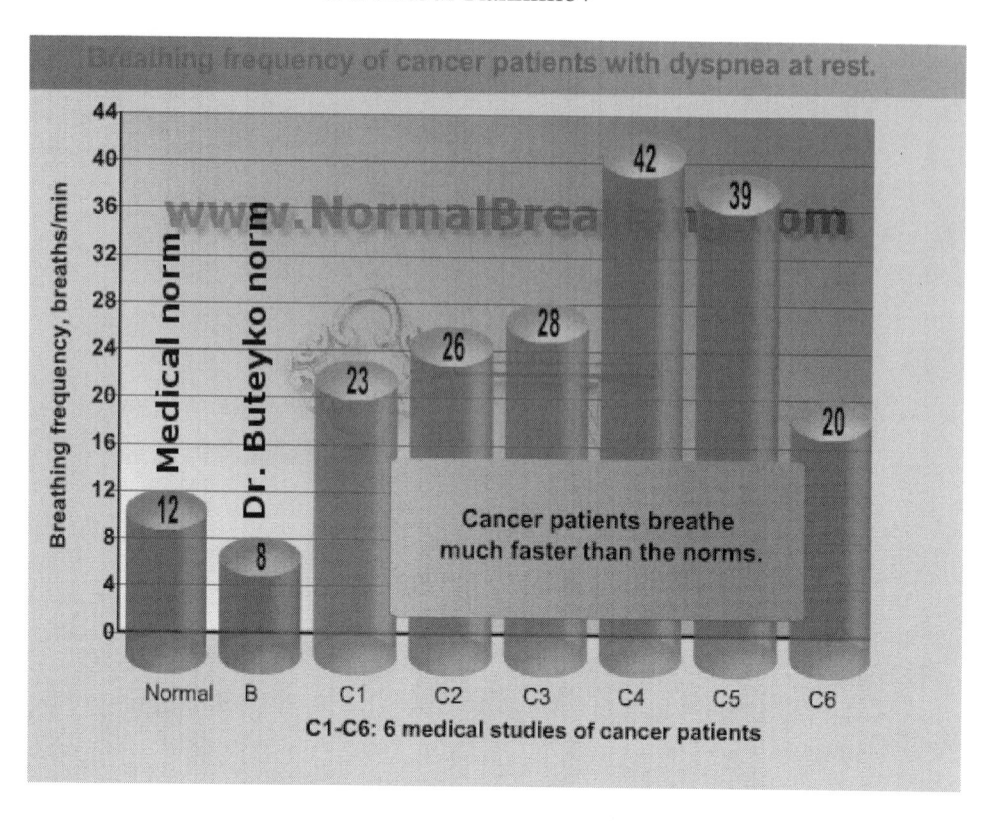

Breathing frequency of cancer patients with dyspnea at rest.

[Chart: Breathing frequency, breaths/min — Normal (Medical norm): 12; B (Dr. Buteyko norm): 8; C1: 23; C2: 26; C3: 28; C4: 42; C5: 39; C6: 20. C1-C6: 6 medical studies of cancer patients. Cancer patients breathe much faster than the norms.]

The same results for Rf (respiratory frequency) are provided in this table.

Condition	N.of people	Rf	References
Medical norm	-	12	Medical textbooks
Dr. Buteyko norm	-	8	Buteyko, 1991
Cancer with dyspnea	10	23	Bruera et al, 1993
Cancer with dyspnea	9	26	Mazzocato et al, 1999
Cancer with dyspnea	20	28	Coyne et al, 2002
Cancer with dyspnea	11	42	Clemens et al, 2007
Cancer with dyspnea	14	39	Clemens et al, 2008
Cancer with dyspnea	20	20	Travers et al, 2008
Cancer	20	19	Travers et al, 2008

Note that some of these studies investigated patients with metastatic cancer and terminally sick cancer patients who are often given morphine during last weeks of their lives in order to reduce pain and suffering. Morphine is a powerful respiratory suppressant and can dramatically reduce minute ventilation and Rf. These factors make results for cancer patients different, but in each and every case we observe that they have very fast breathing up to about 2-3 times faster than the official medical norm.

Ukrainian medical doctor Sergey Paschenko measured CO_2 content in the expired air or so called end-tidal CO_2 in 120 women with metastatic breast cancer (Paschenko, 2001). End-tidal CO_2 concentrations are generally very close to the arterial CO_2 concentrations. The average value for end-tidal CO_2 in these cancer patients was about 2.9%, while the official medical norm is about 5.3% that corresponds to 40 mm Hg at sea level.

This study directly confirms the results of all previous studies: **People with cancer have abnormally low CO2 levels in their lungs and arterial blood due to too heavy breathing at rest.**

References

Buteyko KP, *Method of voluntary elimination of deep breathing* [in Russian], in *Buteyko method. Its application in medical practice*, ed. by K.P. Buteyko, 2nd ed., 1991, Titul, Odessa, p.148-165.

Bruera E, MacEachern T, Ripamonti C, Hanson J, *Subcutaneous morphine for dyspnea in cancer patients*, Ann Intern Med. 1993; 119: p. 906-907.

Clemens KE, Klaschik E, *Symptomatic therapy of dyspnea with strong opioids and its effect on ventilation in palliative care patients*, J Pain Symptom Management 2007 Apr; 33(4): p.473-481.

Clemens KE, Klaschik E, *Effect of hydromorphone on ventilation in palliative care patients with dyspnea*, Support Care Cancer. 2008 Jan; 16(1): p.93-99. Epub 2007 Oct 11.

Coyne PJ, Viswanathan R, Smith TJ, *Nebulized fentanyl citrate improves patients' perception of breathing, respiratory rate, and oxygen saturation in dyspnea*, J Pain Symptom Manage 2002; 23: p.157–160.

Mazzocato C, Buclin T, Rapin CH, *The effects of morphine on dyspnea and ventilatory function in elderly patients with advanced cancer: a randomized double-blind controlled trial*, Annals of Oncology. 1999 Dec; 10(12): p.1511-1514.

Paschenko S, *Study of application of the reduced breathing method in a combined treatment of breast cancer* [in Russian], Oncology (Kiev, Ukraine) 2001, v. 3, No.1, p. 77-78.

Travers J, Dudgeon DJ, Amjadi K, McBride I, Dillon K, Laveneziana P, Ofir D, Webb KA, O'Donnell DE, *Mechanisms of exertional dyspnea in patients with cancer*, J Appl Physiol 2008 Jan; 104(1): p.57-66.

3. Effects of overbreathing (hyperventilation)

We found that people with cancer breathe too much air at rest. Are there any problems with overbreathing? While most people assume that deep breathing or breathing more air is beneficial for health and would mean more O2 in body cells, hundreds of medical research studies found that hyperventilation causes many adverse reactions and no benefits. First of all, as we discussed above, breathing more air does not increase blood oxygenation in any significant degree. Let us consider other effects of chronic overbreathing (or chronic hyperventilation) on the human organism.

If a healthy person with normal breathing starts to breathe more or deeper than the norms, what are the initial effects? There are following consequences:
- More CO2 is removed from the lungs with each breath and therefore the level of CO2 in the airways and lungs immediately decreases.

- In 1-2 minutes, the CO2 level falls below the norm in the arterial blood.
- In 3-5 minutes, due to CO2 diffusion from tissues, most cells of the body (including vital organs and muscles) experience lowered CO2 concentrations.
- In 15-20 minutes, the CO2 level in the brain is below the norm due to a slower diffusion rate caused by the blood-brain barrier.

3.1 Vasoconstriction and reduced blood flow are caused by low CO2 in the arterial blood

Dozens of independent physiological studies found that hypocapnia (low CO2 concentration in the arterial blood) decreased the blood flow for circulation for the following organs:

- brain (Fortune et al, 1995; Karlsson et al, 1994; Liem et al, 1995; Macey et al, 2007; Santiago & Edelman, 1986; Starling & Evans, 1968; Tsuda et al, 1987)
- heart (Coetzee et al, 1984; Foëx et al, 1979; Karlsson et al, 1994; Okazaki et al, 1991; Okazaki et al, 1992; Wexels et al, 1985)
- liver (Dutton et al, 1976; Fujita et al, 1989; Hughes et al, 1979; Okazaki, 1989)
- kidneys (Karlsson et al, 1994; Okazaki, 1989)
- spleen (Karlsson et al, 1994)
- colon (Gilmour et al, 1980).

What is the physiological mechanism of the reduced blood flow to vital organs? CO2 is a dilator of blood vessels (arteries and arterioles). Arteries and arterioles have their own tiny smooth muscles that can constrict or dilate (relax) depending on CO2 concentrations. When we breathe more, CO2 level in the arterial blood decreases, blood vessels constrict and vital organs (like the brain, heart, kidneys, liver, stomach, spleen, colon, etc.) get less blood supply.

Dr. Artour Rakhimov

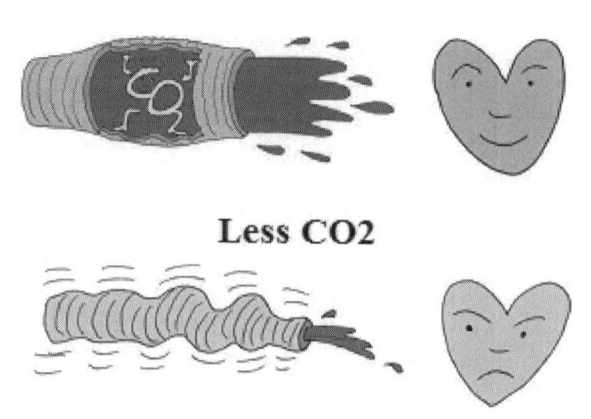

Less CO2

This effect of vasoconstriction is noticeable or detectable even for very small decrease in arterial CO2. This is because CO2 is a very potent vasodilator. Some studies claim that CO2 is a more powerful vasodilator than any chemical drug. For example, medical doctors from the Department of Anesthesia, Armed Forces Hospital, in Riyadh (Saudi Arabia) suggested that "*Carbon dioxide, a most potent cerebral vasodilator...*" (Djurberg et al, 1998).

Dilation of blood vessels means more O2, glucose, and other vital nutrients and chemicals for all organs of the human body. Breathing more air causes constriction of blood vessels. This slows down delivery of all these key chemicals to organs and tissues of the body.

Since all people with cancer are heavy breathers, they naturally have reduced blood flow and reduced oxygen delivery to all vital organs and tissues.

Low CO2 increases pulse

Numerous studies have found that when cancer advances, it is very common for sufferers to have elevated heart rates or pulse. There are even statistical data claiming that lower heart rates and lower respiratory rates in people with advanced forms of cancer are predictors of their better survival. However, we can show that these two parameters relate to each other.

In fact, during the first decades of the 20th century, the respiratory and cardiovascular systems were not divided yet. The leading physiologists and main medical textbooks of the time studied the **cardiorespiratory system** as one mainly due to the intimate links between the systems How are they linked? While the effects and interactions between them are numerous, there is one main relationship that is based on the effects of CO2 to dilate blood vessels.

The state of arteries and arterioles controls the total resistance to the systemic blood flow in the human body. Hence, when the arterial CO2 is normal or high, the arteries and arterioles are dilated, and it is easy for the heart to push blood for the total circulation. However, low CO2 or hypocapnia increases total resistance and the strain on the heart. Therefore, breathing patterns directly participate in regulation of the heart rate.

The father of cardiorespiratory physiology, Yale University Professor Yandell Henderson (1873-1944) was the author of the first medical textbooks on respiration. He knew about this CO2 effect on the heart rate. During one of his physiological projects, he performed experiments with anaesthetized dogs on mechanical ventilation. The results were described in his article "*Acapnia and shock. - I. Carbon dioxide as a factor in the regulation of the heart rate*". In this 1908 article, published in the *American Journal of Physiology*, he noticed, "*... we were enabled to regulate the heart to any desired rate from 40 or fewer up to 200 or more beats per minute. The method was very simple. It depended on the manipulation of the hand bellows with which artificial respiration was administered... As the pulmonary ventilation increased or diminished the heart rate was correspondingly accelerated or retarded*" (p.127, Henderson, 1908).

Note that the effects of changes in breathing on heart rate, as well as blood pressure, are individual in a short run. However, when there are chronic changes in automatic breathing patterns in the direction of hyperventilation, nearly all people develop higher pulse. Is there any significance in these variables for cancer patients?

Generally, when doctors try to identify the key factors that predict survival of cancer patients, they choose various blood parameters that require special laboratory testing, dyspnea score, presence of edema, delirium, loss of appetite, and some other variables.

However, in one study conducted by Spanish researchers, they decided to use those factors that can be easily measured. The title of their study was "*Palliative performance status, heart rate and respiratory rate as predictive factors of survival time in terminally ill cancer patients*" (Sánchez et al, 2006). They tested 98 patients, and in the conclusions wrote, "*The median survival was 32 days. In the multivariate analysis, three independent variables were identified: Palliative Performance Score of 50 or under, heart rate of 100/minute or more, and respiratory rate of 24/minute or more. The variables that were found to be prognostic in our study are objective, easy, and quick to measure, and do not require that the professional have special training or experience*".

Therefore, it is logical to expect that if people with cancer slow down their breathing closer or back to the medical norms, they can expect reduced average respiratory frequencies (slower breathing) and decreased heart rates, at the same time. Furthermore, these numbers for the heart rate and breathing frequency are in complete agreement with parameters for the terminally sick people that are provided by the Buteyko Table of Health Zones.

This is quite consistent with what Dr. Buteyko discovered in the 1960's after analyzing hundreds of subjects of varying degrees of health. He suggested the use of a system utilizing 12 health zones with each zone corresponding to their own average cardiorespiratory parameters. The last zone of his proposed system corresponds to patients whose heart rates were more than 100 beats/min and whose respiratory rates were beyond 24 breaths/min. This is the zone where terminally sick patients qualify, and it is consistent with the numbers which the study of Sanchez concluded with. We will discuss this Buteyko Table further below:

We can now conclude that since both breathing frequency and pulse are factors for survival, easier breathing is something that each every cancer patient needs.

Effects of overbreathing on the brain

Advancing cancer has a profound effect on emotional, mental, and spiritual lives of patients. Depression, anxiety, confusion, insomnia, delirium, and many other problems become more and more common in people with advancing cancer. Can we anticipate all these problems? Yes, if we know that they breathing becomes faster and heavier. If a healthy person starts to hyperventilate or breathe very heavy and fast at rest, what are the effects on the brain? As a result of voluntary hyperventilation, this person would feel dizzy and could easily faint or pass out in about 2-3 minutes.

What are the causes of dizziness and fainting? Many people believe that too much oxygen in the brain is the cause of these effects, and we already know that very small and slow normal breathing results in having the near ideal oxygenation of the arterial blood (about 98-99%). We cannot increase blood oxygenation by taking a deep breath or many deep breaths. The illustration below shows a brain scan undergoing two conditions: during normal breathing and after 1 minute of voluntary hyperventilation. The red color represents the most O2, dark blue the least. This illustration shows that a person's brain oxygenation is reduced by about 40% or to nearly just half simply by hyperventilation (Litchfield, 2003).

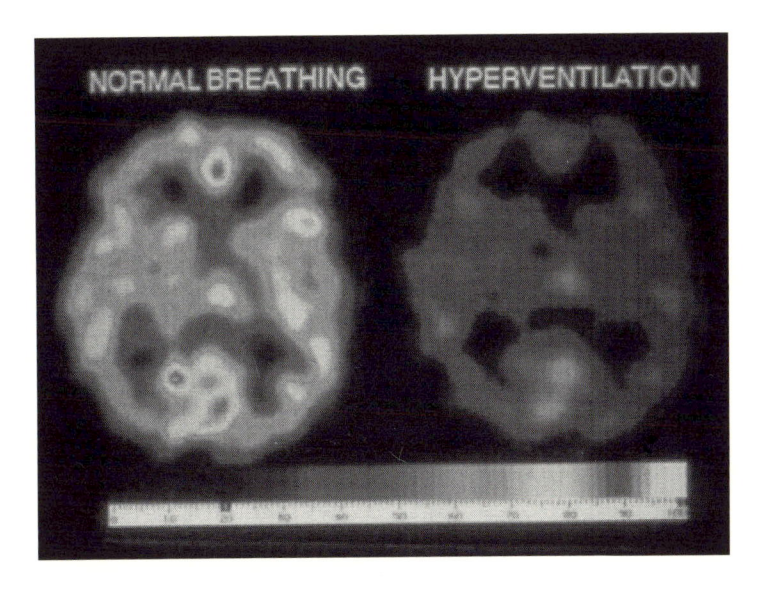

This result is quoted in medical textbooks (e.g., Starling & Evans, 1968) since the effect is well documented and has been confirmed by dozens of professional medical experiments. According to the Handbook of Physiology (Santiago & Edelman, 1986), cerebral blood flow decreases by about 2% for every mm Hg decrease in CO_2 pressure.

Since cancer patients have heavy breathing all the time, it is sensible to say that they suffer from reduced brain oxygenation. In addition, there are negative effects of low CO_2 on nerve cells that we are going to discuss below.

References

Coetzee A, Holland D, Foëx P, Ryder A, Jones L, *The effect of hypocapnia on coronary blood flow and myocardial function in the dog*, Anesthesia and Analgesia 1984 Nov; 63(11): p. 991-997.

Dutton R, Levitzky M, Berkman R, *Carbon dioxide and liver blood flow*, Bull Eur Physiopathol Respir. 1976 Mar-Apr; 12(2): p. 265-273.

Gilmour DG, Douglas IH, Aitkenhead AR, Hothersall AP, Horton PW, Ledingham IM, *Colon blood flow in the dog: effects of changes in arterial carbon dioxide tension*, Cardiovasc Res 1980 Jan; 14(1): 11-20.

Djurberg HG, Tjan GT, Al Moutaery KR, *Enhanced catheter propagation with hypercapnia during superselective cerebral catherisation*, Neuroradiology. 1998 Jul;40(7):466-8.

Foëx P, Ryder WA, *Effect of CO2 on the systemic and coronary circulations and on coronary sinus blood gas tensions*, Bull Eur Physiopathol Respir 1979 Jul-Aug; 15(4): p.625-638.

Fortune JB, Feustel PJ, deLuna C, Graca L, Hasselbarth J, Kupinski AM, *Cerebral blood flow and blood volume in response to O2 and CO2 changes in normal humans*, J Trauma. 1995 Sep; 39(3): p. 463-471.

Fujita Y, Sakai T, Ohsumi A, Takaori M, *Effects of hypocapnia and hypercapnia on splanchnic circulation and hepatic function in the beagle*, Anesthesia and Analgesia 1989 Aug; 69(2): p. 152-157.

Hashimoto K, Okazaki K, Okutsu Y, *The effects of hypocapnia and hypercapnia on tissue surface PO2 in hemorrhaged dogs* [Article in Japanese], Masui 1989 Oct; 38(10): p. 1271-1274.

Henderson Y, *Acapnia and shock. - I. Carbon dioxide as a factor in the regulation of the heart rate*, American Journal of Physiology 1908, 21: p. 126-156.

Hughes RL, Mathie RT, Fitch W, Campbell D, *Liver blood flow and oxygen consumption during hypocapnia and IPPV in the greyhound*, J Appl Physiol. 1979 Aug; 47(2): p. 290-295.

Karlsson T, Stjernström EL, Stjernström H, Norlén K, Wiklund L, *Central and regional blood flow during hyperventilation. An experimental study in the pig*, Acta Anaesthesiol Scand. 1994 Feb; 38(2): p.180-186.

Liem KD, Kollée LA, Hopman JC, De Haan AF, Oeseburg B, *The influence of arterial carbon dioxide on cerebral oxygenation and haemodynamics during ECMO in normoxaemic and hypoxaemic piglets*, Acta Anaesthesiol Scand Suppl. 1995; 107: p.157-164.

Litchfield PM, *A brief overview of the chemistry of respiration and the breathing heart wave*, California Biofeedback, 2003 Spring, 19(1).

Macey PM, Woo MA, Harper RM, *Hyperoxic brain effects are normalized by addition of CO2*, PLoS Med. 2007 May; 4(5): p. e173.

McArdle WD, Katch FI, Katch VL, *Essentials of exercise physiology* (2-nd edition); Lippincott, Williams and Wilkins, London 2000.

Okazaki K, Okutsu Y, Fukunaga A, *Effect of carbon dioxide (hypocapnia and hypercapnia) on tissue blood flow and oxygenation of liver, kidneys and skeletal muscle in the dog*, Masui 1989 Apr, 38 (4): p. 457-464.

Okazaki K, Hashimoto K, Okutsu Y, Okumura F, *Effect of arterial carbon dioxide tension on regional myocardial tissue oxygen tension in the dog* [Article in Japanese], Masui 1991 Nov; 40(11): p. 1620-1624.

Okazaki K, Hashimoto K, Okutsu Y, Okumura F, *Effect of carbon dioxide (hypocapnia and hypercapnia) on regional myocardial tissue oxygen tension in dogs with coronary stenosis* [Article in Japanese], Masui 1992 Feb; 41(2): p. 221-224.

de Miguel Sánchez C, Elustondo SG, Estirado A, Sánchez FV, de la Rasilla Cooper CG, Romero AL, Otero A, Olmos LG, *Palliative performance status, heart rate and respiratory rate as predictive factors of survival time in terminally ill cancer patients,* J Pain Symptom Manage. 2006 Jun;31(6):485-92.

Santiago TV & Edelman NH, *Brain blood flow and control of breathing*, in *Handbook of Physiology, Section 3: The respiratory system*, vol. II, ed. by AP Fishman. American Physiological Society, Betheda, Maryland, 1986, p. 163-179.

Starling E & Lovatt EC, *Principles of human physiology*, 14-th ed., 1968, Lea & Febiger, Philadelphia.

Tsuda Y, Kimura K, Yoneda S, Hartmann A, Etani H, Hashikawa K, Kamada T, *Effect of hypocapnia on cerebral oxygen metabolism and blood flow in ischemic cerebrovascular disorders*, Eur Neurol. 1987; 27(3): p.155-163.

Wexels JC, Myhre ES, Mjøs OD, *Effects of carbon dioxide and pH on myocardial blood-flow and metabolism in the dog*, Clin Physiol. 1985 Dec; 5(6): p.575-588.

3.2 Low CO2 results in the suppressed Bohr effect

There is an additional negative effect of low CO2 on oxygen delivery. We now know that hypocapnia decreases blood supply to all vital organs. Why do hemoglobin cells or red blood cells release oxygen in the tissues, but not in the arteries, or arterioles, or veins? Why is more O2 released in those tissues of the human body that use more energy? For example, the heart, due to its constant work, gets more O2 than those muscles that are at rest.
The answer is in the Bohr's law (or Bohr effect). The Bohr effect was first described in 1904 by the Danish physiologist Christian Bohr. He was the father of famous physicist Niels Bohr. Christian Bohr discovered that due to higher CO2 content in tissues and capillaries (more acidic environment than in arteries and arterioles), hemoglobin is bound to oxygen with less affinity. Hence, oxygen is released in tissues due to higher CO2 levels in those tissues.

CO₂ releases O₂ from blood

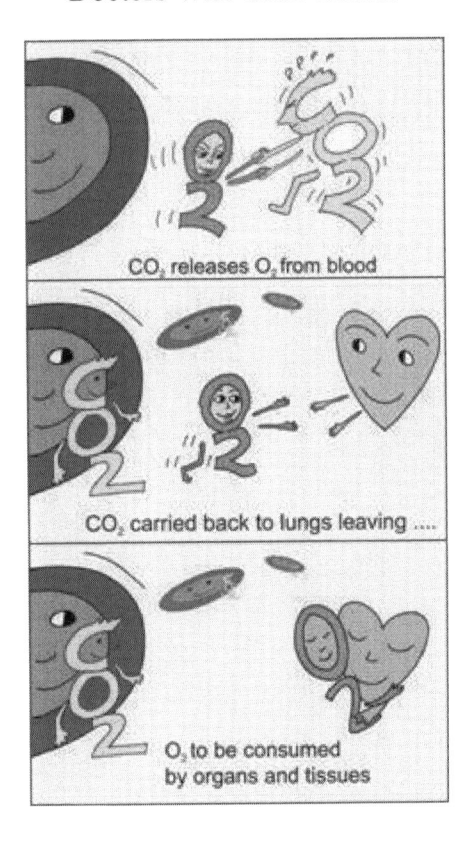

CO₂ carried back to lungs leaving....

O₂ to be consumed by organs and tissues

There are many modern professional investigations devoted to various aspects of the Bohr effect (e.g., Braumann et al, 1982; Böning et al, 1975; Bucci et al, 1985; Carter et al, 1985; diBella et al, 1986; Dzhagarov et al, 1996; Grant et al, 1982; Grubb et al, 1979; Gersonde et al, 1986; Hlastala & Woodson, 1983; Jensen, 2004; Kister et al, 1988; Kobayashi et al, 1989; Lapennas, 1983; Matthew et al, 1979; Meyer et al, 1978; Tyuma, 1984; Winslow et al, 1985).

Hyperventilation causes reduced CO2 tissue tension, and this leads to reduced O2 release and reduced oxygen tension in tissues (Aarnoudse et al, 1981; Monday & Tétreault, 1980; Gottstein et al, 1976). In simple terms, low absolute CO2 values prevent effective release of oxygen by red blood cells in tissues of the human body, and the blood carries oxygen away from tissues when there are no CO2.

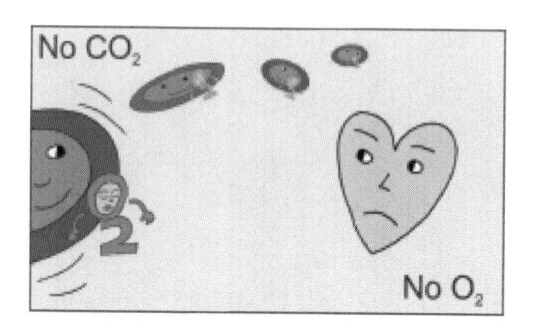

In order to improve the release of oxygen by red blood cells in tissues, cancer patients require normal (or even slightly above the norm) arterial CO2 values.

References

Aarnoudse JG, Oeseburg B, Kwant G, Zwart A, Zijlstra WG, Huisjes HJ, *Influence of variations in pH and PCO2 on scalp tissue oxygen tension and carotid arterial oxygen tension in the fetal lamb*, Biol Neonate 1981; 40(5-6): p. 252-263.

Braumann KM, Böning D, Trost F, *Bohr effect and slope of the oxygen dissociation curve after physical training*, J Appl Physiol. 1982 Jun; 52(6): p. 1524-1529.

Böning D, Schwiegart U, Tibes U, Hemmer B, *Influences of exercise and endurance training on the oxygen dissociation curve of blood under in vivo and in vitro conditions*, Eur J Appl Physiol Occup Physiol. 1975; 34(1): p. 1-10.

Bucci E, Fronticelli C, *Anion Bohr effect of human hemoglobin*, Biochemistry. 1985 Jan 15; 24(2): p. 371-376. Carter AM, Grønlund J, *Contribution of the Bohr effect to the fall in fetal PO2 caused by maternal alkalosis*, J Perinat Med. 1985; 13(4): p.185-191.

diBella G, Scandariato G, Suriano O, Rizzo A, *Oxygen affinity and Bohr effect responses to 2,3-diphosphoglycerate in equine and human blood*, Res Vet Sci. 1996 May; 60(3): p. 272-275.

Dzhagarov BM, Kruk NN, *The alkaline Bohr effect: regulation ofthnded hemoglobin Hb(O2)3* [Article in Russian] Biofizika. 1996 May-Jun; 41(3): p. 606-612.

Gersonde K, Sick H, Overkamp M, Smith KM, Parish DW, *Bohr effect in monomeric insect haemoglobins controlled by O2 off-rate and modulated by haem-rotational disorder*, Eur J Biochem. 1986 Jun 2; 157(2): p. 393-404.

Grant BJ, *Influence of Bohr-Haldane effect on steady-state gas exchange*, J Appl Physiol. 1982 May; 52(5): p. 1330-1337.

Grubb B, Jones JH, Schmidt-Nielsen K, *Avian cerebral blood flow: influence of the Bohr effect on oxygen supply*, Am J Physiol. 1979 May; 236(5): p. H744-749.

Gottstein U, Zahn U, Held K, Gabriel FH, Textor T, Berghoff W, *Effect of hyperventilation on cerebral blood flow and metabolism in man; continuous monitoring of arterio-cerebral venous glucose differences* (author's transl) [Article in German], Klin Wochenschr. 1976 Apr 15; 54(8): p. 373-381.

Hlastala MP, Woodson RD, *Bohr effect data for blood gas calculations*, J Appl Physiol. 1983 Sep; 55(3): p. 1002-1007.

Jensen FB, *Red blood cell pH, the Bohr effect, and other oxygenation-linked phenomena in blood O2 and CO2 transport*, Acta Physiol Scand. 2004 Nov; 182(3): p. 215-227.

Kister J, Marden MC, Bohn B, Poyart C, *Functional properties of hemoglobin in human red cells: II. Determination of the Bohr effect*, Respir Physiol. 1988 Sep; 73(3): p. 363-378.

Kobayashi H, Pelster B, Piiper J, Scheid P, *Significance of the Bohr effect for tissue oxygenation in a model with counter-current blood flow*, Respir Physiol. 1989 Jun; 76(3): p. 277-288.

Lapennas GN, *The magnitude of the Bohr coefficient: optimal for oxygen delivery*, Respir Physiol. 1983 Nov; 54(2): p.161-172.

Matthew JB, Hanania GI, Gurd FR, *Electrostatic effects in hemoglobin: Bohr effect and ionic strength dependence of individual groups*, Biochemistry. 1979 May 15; 18(10): p.1928-1936.

Meyer M, Holle JP, Scheid P, *Bohr effect induced by CO2 and fixed acid at various levels of O2 saturation in duck blood*, Pflugers Arch. 1978 Sep 29; 376(3): p. 237-240.

Monday LA, Tétreault L, *Hyperventilation and vertigo*, Laryngoscope 1980 Jun; 90(6 Pt 1): p.1003-1010.

Tyuma I, *The Bohr effect and the Haldane effect in human hemoglobin*, Jpn J Physiol. 1984; 34(2): p.205-216.

Winslow RM, Monge C, Winslow NJ, Gibson CG, Whittembury J, *Normal whole blood Bohr effect in Peruvian natives of high altitude*, Respir Physiol. 1985 Aug; 61(2): p. 197-208.

3.3 Less oxygen for cells

Summarizing these above-discussed physiological CO2 effects, we conclude:

1. Hyperventilation cannot increase O2 content in the arterial blood to any significant degree (normal hemoglobin saturation is about 98-99%), but it instead reduces CO2 concentrations in all cells and the blood.
2. Hypocapnia (or CO2 deficiency) leads to constriction of blood vessels, and that reduces blood supply to vital organs of the human body.
3. Hypocapnia (or CO2 deficiency) also leads to the suppressed Bohr effect that causes further reduction in oxygen delivery.
4. Hyperventilation causes low O2 levels in cells.

Hence, the more cancer patient breathes, the less oxygen is provided for all vital organs. This generates free radicals, causes more problems with chronic inflammation, and fueling advance of cancer.

The discussed effects of low CO2 due to hyperventilation oxygen transport are summarized in these two graphs.

Normal gas exchanges

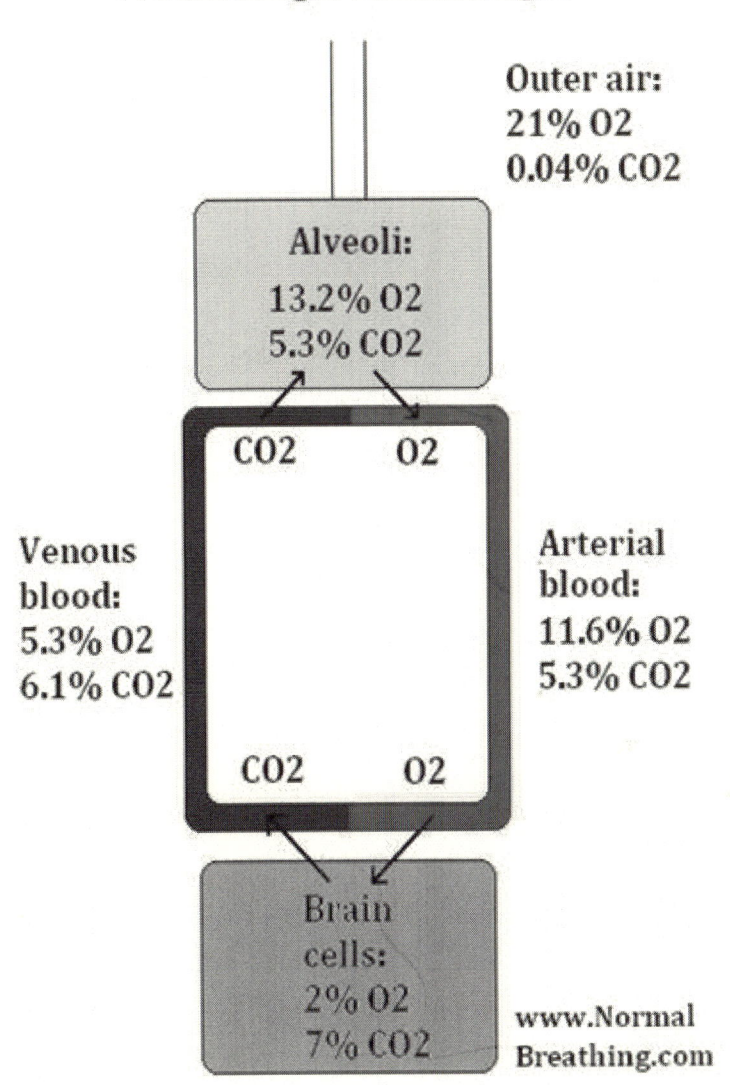

Outer air:
21% O2
0.04% CO2

Alveoli:
13.2% O2
5.3% CO2

CO2   O2

Venous blood:
5.3% O2
6.1% CO2

Arterial blood:
11.6% O2
5.3% CO2

CO2   O2

Brain cells:
2% O2
7% CO2

www.NormalBreathing.com

Effects of hyperventilation on circulation and normal gas exchange

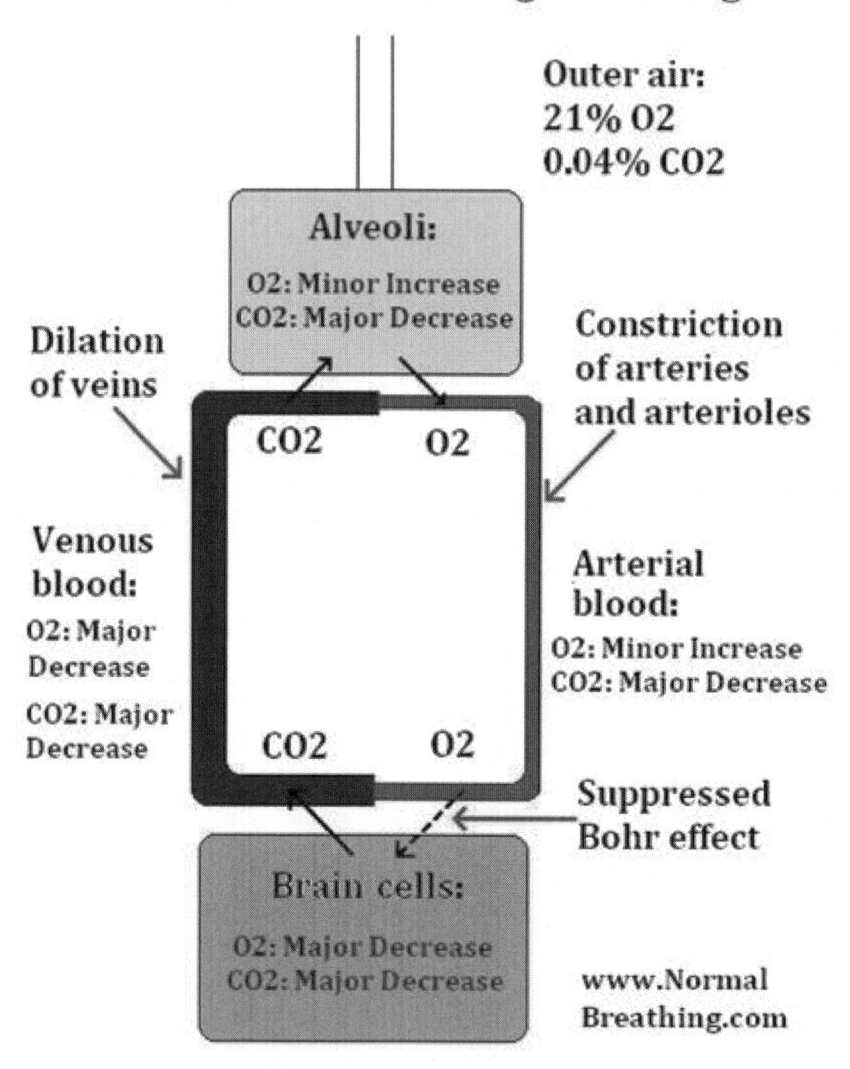

Outer air: 21% O2, 0.04% CO2

Alveoli:
O2: Minor Increase
CO2: Major Decrease

Dilation of veins

Constriction of arteries and arterioles

Venous blood:
O2: Major Decrease
CO2: Major Decrease

Arterial blood:
O2: Minor Increase
CO2: Major Decrease

Suppressed Bohr effect

Brain cells:
O2: Major Decrease
CO2: Major Decrease

www.NormalBreathing.com

3.4 Other effects of low arterial CO2

Among other effects of low arterial CO2 are:
- **abnormal excitability and irritability of nerve cells** (e.g., Brown, 1953; Krnjevic, 1965; Balestrino & Somjen, 1988; Huttunen et al, 1999)

- **irritable state of muscles or worsened muscular tension** (Brown, 1953; Hudlicka, 1973)

- **bronchospasm** or reduced diameter of airways causing wheezing, dyspnea and sensations of breathlessness and suffocation (Sterling, 1968)

- **abnormalities with ions in blood plasma and other bodily fluids** (Carryer, 1947)

- **innumerable abnormalities involving synthesis of amino acids, carbohydrates, hormones, lipids (fats), messengers, cells of the immune system, etc**.

Dr. Brown in his article *"Physiological effects of hyperventilation"* analyzed almost 300 professional studies. He wrote *"Studies designed to determine the effects produced by hyperventilation on nerve and muscle have been consistent in their finding on increased irritability"* (Brown, 1953). Other authors (e.g., Balestrino & Somjen, 1988; Huttunen et al, 1999) also concluded that increased CO2 pressure generally reduces cortical excitability, while hyperventilation *"leads to spontaneous and asynchronous firing of cortical neurons"* (Huttunen et. al., 1999).

These are exceptionally important conclusions related to understanding of psychological and mental problems in people with advanced cancer. Their heavy breathing is the cause of their depression, chronic fatigue (i.e., hypoxia in muscle cells), anxiety, confusion, sleeping problems, and many other abnormalities related to reduced quality of life.

References

Balestrino M, Somjen GG, *Concentration of carbon dioxide, interstitial pH and synaptic transmission in hippocampal formation of the rat*, J Physiol 1988, 396: p. 247-266.

Brown EB, *Physiological effects of hyperventilation*, Physiol Reviews 1953 Oct, 33 (4): p. 445-471.

Carryer HM, *Hyperventilation syndrome*, Med Clin North Amer 1947, 31: p. 845.

Hudlicka O, *Muscle blood flow*, 1973, Swets&Zeitlinger, Amsterdam.

Huttunen J, Tolvanen H, Heinonen E, Voipio J, Wikstrom H, Ilmoniemi RJ, Hari R, Kaila K, *Effects of voluntary hyperventilation on cortical sensory responses*. Electroencephalographic and magnetoencephalographic studies, Exp Brain Res 1999, 125(3): p. 248-254.

Krnjevic K, Randic M and Siesjo B, *Cortical CO2 tension and neuronal excitability*, J of Physiol 1965, 176: p. 105-122.

Sterling GM, *The mechanism of bronchoconstriction due to hypocapnia in man*, Clin Sci 1968 Apr; 34(2): p. 277-285.

3.5 Are there any benefits from hyperventilation?

In some cases, a person can visually observe effects of breathing on blood flow. For example, if you get a small bleeding cut or a wound, you can deliberately hyperventilate and see that overbreathing will help to stop the bleeding. As an alternative, you can perform breath holding, breathe less and accumulate more CO_2. Your blood losses will increase.

Many dental surgeons know about this effect and they advise their clients to breathe more during and after dental surgeries to prevent excessive blood losses. The same can be done for brain traumas and other accidents involving bleeding. It is natural for humans and other animals to breathe heavily in such conditions of stress and pain. Hence, hyperventilation can be life-saving in such cases of severe bleeding.

Why did Nature provide us with these physiological reactions caused by hyperventilation? Breathing is closely connected with blood flow to all vital organs, sensitivity of the immune system, permeability of cellular membranes, and many other key functions. It becomes heavier as a natural response when vital organs such as the brain, heart, stomach, kidney, liver, etc undergo chemical, viral, bacteriological or other similar stresses, or inflammation or injury.

Hyperventilation thus helps to prevent:

- excessive bleeding (as in cases of open injuries, cuts, bruises, etc.)

- quick spread of bacterial and viral infections

- excessive amounts of toxic products in the blood from injured, infected, or polluted tissues

- damage to vital cleansing organs (e.g., liver and kidneys) due to their possible toxic overload.

All these preventive effects from hyperventilation can save the life of a person in the short run. At the same time, it is not normal to be in a state of stress and chronic hyperventilation all the time. Our breathing, if there is no emergency, should be normal. This ensures normal O_2 delivery and normalization of hundreds of other essential bodily processes.

4. Why cancer is common now?

4.1 Breathing in ordinary people

Cancer has been known for thousands of years. We can read its description in manuscripts coming from ancient Egypt. However, there was an explosion in cancer rates during the 20th century. Previously, the number of people affected by cancer was many tens of times smaller. What are the causes of this increase? Why is that nearly any modern person, as oncologist and scientists say, is prone to cancer?

As you may remember from the previous parts of this book, cancer is controlled by cellular oxygen levels, and people with cancer have low body O2 due to their heavy breathing. One of the above-mentioned studies found that cancer patients had about 12 liters per minute for their breathing at rest or about twice more than the norm. However, contemporary people, in average, are not different. Consider this graph that represents minute ventilation rates in normal people over the span of last 80 years.

Hyperventilation: Present in Over 90% of Modern Normals

This information is based on 24 published medical studies

Norm	1929	1939	1939	1950	1980s	90-96	1997	98-99	2000s
6	4.9	5.3	4.6	6.9	7.8	12	11	12	12

Minute Ventilation, liters per min

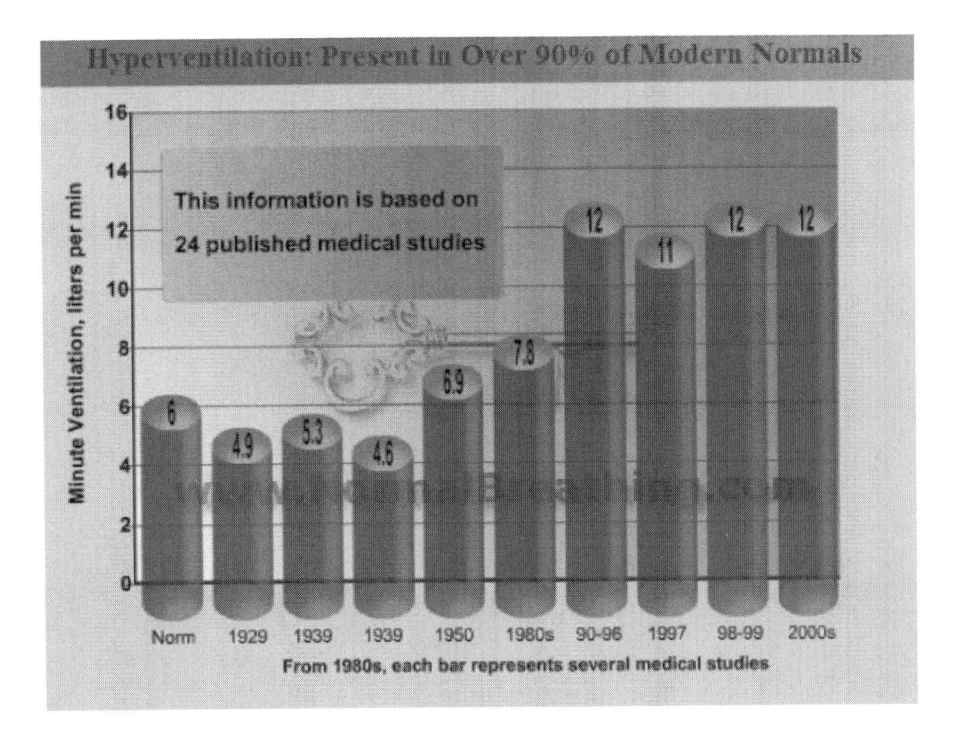

From 1980s, each bar represents several medical studies

The graph represents results of 24 medical studies (from 1929 until 2007). It tells us that, during the 1920s and 30s, breathing rates of ordinary people were even less than normal. However, during the 1990s and later, ordinary people breathe about 2 times more air than the medical norm, or about the same as people with cancer. Here are the more detailed results presented on the graph.

Condition	Minute ventilation	Age	N. of subjects	References
Healthy Subjects	6-7 L/min	-	>400	Results of 14 studies
Normal breathing	6	-	-	Medical textbooks
Normal subjects	4.9	-	5	Griffith et al, 1929
Normal males	5.3±0.1	27-43	46	Shock et al, 1939
Normal females	4.6±0.1	27-43	40	Shock et al, 1939
Normal subjects	6.9±0.9	-	100	Matheson et al, 1950
Normal subjects	9.1±4.5	31±7	11	Kassabian et al, 1982
Normal subjects	8.1±2.1	42±14	11	D'Alonzo et al, 1987
Normal subjects	6.3±2.2	-	12	Pain et al, 1988
Normal males	13±3	40 (av.)	12	Clague et al, 1994
Normal subjects	9.2±2.5	34±7	13	Radwan et al, 1995
Normal subjects	15±4	28-34	12	Dahan et al, 1995
Normal subjects	12±4	55±10	43	Clark et al, 1995
Normal subjects	12±2	41±2	10	Tantucci et al, 1996
Normal subjects*	11±3	53±11	24	Clark et al, 1997

Condition	Minute ventilation	Age	N. of subjects	Reference
Normal subjects	8.1±0.4	34±2	63	Meessen et al, 1997
Normal females	9.9	20-28	23	Han et al, 1997
Normal males	15	20-28	47	Han et al, 1997
Normal females	10	29-60	42	Han et al, 1997
Normal males	11	29-62	42	Han et al, 1997
Normal subjects	13±3	36±6	10	Tantucci et al, 1997
Normal subjects	12±1	65±2	10	Epstein et al, 1996
Normal subjects	12±1	12-69	20	Bowler et al, 1998
Normal subjects	10±6	39±4	20	DeLorey et al, 1999
Normal seniors	12±4	70±3	14	DeLorey et al, 1999
Normal elderly[+]	14±3	88±2	11	DeLorey et al, 1999
Normal subjects	17±1	41±2	15	Tantucci et al, 2001
Normal subjects	10±0.5	-	10	Bell et al, 2005
Normal subjects	8.5±1.2	30±8	69	Narkiewicz, 2006
Normal females	10±0.4	-	11	Ahuja et al, 2007
Normal subjects	12±2	62±2	20	Travers et al, 2008

* For some studies, when the average weight of the subjects was significantly different from 70 kg, minute ventilation was adjusted to the normal weight (70 kg) value.

Note that the results are somewhat inconsistent since there is no strict definition for "normal" or "control" subjects in medical research. Consider a typical medical study. If the organizers of this medical study want to measure the effects of some medication or treatment on a group of people with cancer, the researchers may also select a group of control subjects for comparison. These "control" subjects must be cancer-free. These control subjects are thus called "normal subjects". On the other hand, if these subjects are free from any serious health problem, they are called "healthy subjects".

Many people and researchers say that cancer is caused by toxic chemicals, smoking, pollution, poor diet, lack of exercise, and other factors. I completely agree with these statements, and there are even studies that confirmed these specific relationships. However, we can go beyond these statements since all these lifestyle risk factors makes people to hyperventilate and reduced their body oxygenation. Furthermore, there are other more damaging hidden lifestyle risk factors and other parameters that are not known to most doctors and ordinary people. They relate to sleep, exercise, diet, focal infections, and some other characteristics. All these abnormalities make breathing heavier. Therefore, they all are the driving forces of cancer in modern population.

References for the Tables (in the same order)

Griffith FR, Pucher GW, Brownell KA, Klein JD, Carmer ME, *Studies in human physiology. IV. Vital capacity, respiratory rate and volume, and composition of the expired air.* Am. J. Physiol 1929, vol. 89, p. 555.

Shock NW, Soley MH, *Average Values for Basal Respiratory Functions in Adolescents and Adults*, J. Nutrition, 1939, 18, p. 143.

Matheson HW, Gray JS, *Ventilatory function tests. III Resting ventilation, metabolism, and derived measures*, J Clin Invest 1950 June; 29(6): p. 688–692.

Kassabian J, Miller KD, Lavietes MH, *Respiratory center output and ventilatory timing in patients with acute airway (asthma) and alveolar (pneumonia) disease*, Chest 1982 May; 81(5): p.536-543.

D'Alonzo GE, Gianotti LA, Pohil RL, Reagle RR, DuRee SL, Fuentes F, Dantzker DR, *Comparison of progressive exercise performance of normal subjects and patients with primary pulmonary hypertension*, Chest 1987 Jul; 92(1): p.57-62.

Pain MC, Biddle N, Tiller JW, *Panic disorder, the ventilatory response to carbon dioxide and respiratory variables*, Psychosom Med 1988 Sep-Oct; 50(5): p. 541-548.

Clague JE, Carter J, Coakley J, Edwards RH, Calverley PM, *Respiratory effort perception at rest and during carbon dioxide rebreathing in patients with dystrophia myotonica*, Thorax 1994 Mar; 49(3): p.240-244.

Radwan L, Maszczyk Z, Koziorowski A, Koziej M, Cieslicki J, Sliwinski P, Zielinski J, *Control of breathing in obstructive sleep apnoea and in patients with the overlap syndrome*, Eur Respir J. 1995 Apr; 8(4): p.542-545.

Dahan A, van den Elsen MJ, Berkenbosch A, DeGoede J, Olievier IC, van Kleef JW, *Halothane affects ventilatory afterdischarge in humans*, Br J Anaesth 1995 May; 74(5): p.544-548.

Clark AL, Chua TP, Coats AJ, *Anatomical dead space, ventilatory pattern, and exercise capacity in chronic heart failure*, Br Heart J 1995 Oct; 74(4): p. 377-380.

Tantucci C, Bottini P, Dottorini ML, Puxeddu E, Casucci G, Scionti L, Sorbini CA, *Ventilatory response to exercise in diabetic subjects with autonomic neuropathy*, J Appl Physiol 1996, 81(5): p.1978–1986.

Clark AL, Volterrani M, Swan JW, Coats AJS, *The increased ventilatory response to exercise in chronic heart failure: relation to pulmonary pathology*, Heart 1997; 77: p.138-146.

Meessen NE, van der Grinten CP, Luijendijk SC, Folgering HT, *Breathing pattern during bronchial challenge in humans*, Eur Respir J 1997 May; 10(5): p.1059-1063.

Han JN, Stegen K, Simkens K, Cauberghs M, Schepers R, Van den Bergh O, Clément J, Van de Woestijne KP, *Unsteadiness of breathing in patients with hyperventilation syndrome and anxiety disorders*, Eur Respir J 1997; 10: p. 167–176.

Tantucci C, Scionti L, Bottini P, Dottorini ML, Puxeddu E, Casucci G, Sorbini CA, *Influence of autonomic neuropathy of different severities on the hypercapnic drive to breathing in diabetic patients*, Chest. 1997 Jul; 112(1): 145-153.

Epstein SK, Zilberberg MD; Facoby C, Ciubotaru RL, Kaplan LM, *Response to symptom-limited exercise in patients with the hepatopulmonary syndrome*, Chest 1998; 114; p. 736-741.

Bowler SD, Green A, Mitchell CA, *Buteyko breathing techniques in asthma: a blinded randomised controlled trial*, Med J of Australia 1998; 169: p. 575-578.

DeLorey DS, Babb TG, *Progressive mechanical ventilatory constraints with aging*, Am J Respir Crit Care Med 1999 Jul; 160(1): p.169-177.

Tantucci C, Bottini P, Fiorani C, Dottorini ML, Santeusanio F, Provinciali L, Sorbini CA, Casucci G, *Cerebrovascular reactivity and hypercapnic respiratory drive in diabetic autonomic neuropathy*, J Appl Physiol 2001, 90: p. 889–896.

Bell HJ, Feenstra W, Duffin J, *The initial phase of exercise hyperpnoea in humans is depressed during a cognitive task*, Experimental Physiology 2005 May; 90(3): p.357-365.

Narkiewicz K, van de Borne P, Montano N, Hering D, Kara T, Somers VK, *Sympathetic neural outflow and chemoreflex sensitivity are related to spontaneous breathing rate in normal men*, Hypertension 2006 Jan; 47(1): p.51-55.

Ahuja D, Mateika JH, Diamond MP, Badr MS, *Ventilatory sensitivity to carbon dioxide before and after episodic hypoxia in women treated with testosterone*, J Appl Physiol. 2007 May; 102(5): p.1832-1838.

Travers J, Dudgeon DJ, Amjadi K, McBride I, Dillon K, Laveneziana P, Ofir D, Webb KA, O'Donnell DE, *Mechanisms of exertional dyspnea in patients with cancer*, J Appl Physiol 2008 Jan; 104(1): p.57-66.

4.2 Minute ventilation in healthy people

Some people may argue, "Probably, due to some reasons, all people started to breathe more, and even healthy people have heavy breathing at rest". No, this is not so. According to these 14 medical studies, healthy people still breathe little air.

Condition	Minute ventilation	N. of subjects	References
Normal breathing	6 L/min	-	Medical textbooks
Healthy subjects	7.7 ± 0.3 L/min	19	Douglas et al, 1982
Healthy males	8.4 ± 1.3 L/min	10	Burki, 1984
Healthy males	6.3 L/min	10	Smits et al, 1987
Healthy males	6.1 ± 1.4 L/min	6	Fuller et al, 1987
Healthy subjects	6.1 ± 0.9 L/min	9	Tanaka et al, 1988
Healthy students	7.0 ± 1.0 L/min	10	Turley et al, 1993
Healthy subjects	6.6 ± 0.6 L/min	10	Bengtsson et al, 1994
Healthy subjects	7.0 ± 1.2 L/min	12	Sherman et al, 1996
Healthy subjects	7.0 ± 1.2 L/min	10	Bell et al, 1996
Healthy subjects	6 ± 1 L/min	7	Parreira et al, 1997
Healthy subjects	7.0 ± 1.1 L/min	14	Mancini et al, 1999
Healthy subjects	6.6 ± 1.1 L/min	40	Pinna et al, 2006
Healthy subjects	6.7 ± 0.5 L/min	17	Pathak et al, 2006
Healthy subjects	6.7 ± 0.3 L/min	14	Gujic et al, 2007

**These clinical observations suggest that healthy people have normal breathing and normal body O2 content. Therefore, they cannot develop any types of cancer. As a result, normal breathing is a guaranteed form of protection from cancer and its prevention.
References for the Table (in the same order)**

Douglas NJ, White DP, Pickett CK, Weil JV, Zwillich CW, *Respiration during sleep in normal man*, Thorax. 1982 Nov; 37(11): p.840-844.

Burki NK, *Ventilatory effects of doxapram in conscious human subjects*, Chest 1984 May; 85(5): p.600-604.
Smits P, Schouten J, Thien T, *Respiratory stimulant effects of adenosine in man after caffeine and enprofylline*, Br J Clin Pharmacol. 1987 Dec; 24(6): p.816-819.

Fuller RW, Maxwell DL, Conradson TB, Dixon CM, Barnes PJ, *Circulatory and respiratory effects of infused adenosine in conscious man*, Br J Clin Pharmacol 1987 Sep; 24(3): p.306-317.

Tanaka Y, Morikawa T, Honda Y, *An assessment of nasal functions in control of breathing*, J of Appl Physiol 1988, 65 (4); p.1520-1524.

Turley KR, McBride PJ, Wilmore LH, *Resting metabolic rate measured after subjects spent the night at home vs at a clinic*, Am J of Clin Nutr 1993, 58, p.141-144.

Bengtsson J, Bengtsson A, Stenqvist O, Bengtsson JP, *Effects of hyperventilation on the inspiratory to end- tidal oxygen difference*, British J of Anaesthesia 1994; 73: p. 140-144.

Sherman MS, Lang DM, Matityahu A, Campbell D, *Theophylline improves measurements of respiratory muscle efficiency*, Chest 1996 Dec; 110(6): p. 437-414. Bell SC, Saunders MJ, Elborn JS, Shale DJ, *Resting energy expenditure and oxygen cost of breathing in patients with cystic fibrosis*, Thorax 1996 Feb; 51(2): 126-131.

Parreira VF, Delguste P, Jounieaux V, Aubert G, Dury M, Rodenstein DO, *Effectiveness of controlled and spontaneous modes in nasal two-level positive pressure ventilation in awake and asleep normal subjects*, Chest 1997 Nov 5; 112(5): p.1267-1277.

Mancini M, Filippelli M, Seghieri G, Iandelli I, Innocenti F, Duranti R, Scano G, *Respiratory Muscle Function and Hypoxic Ventilatory Control in Patients With Type I Diabetes*, Chest 1999; 115; p.1553-1562.

Pinna GD, Maestri R, La Rovere MT, Gobbi E, Fanfulla F, *Effect of paced breathing on ventilatory and cardiovascular variability parameters during short-term investigations of autonomic function*, Am J Physiol Heart Circ Physiol. 2006 Jan; 290(1): p.H424-433.

Pathak A, Velez-Roa S, Xhaët O, Najem B, van de Borne P, *Dose-dependent effect of dobutamine on chemoreflex activity in healthy volunteers*, Br J Clin Pharmacol. 2006 Sep; 62(3): p.272-279.

Gujic M, Houssière A, Xhaët O, Argacha JF, Denewet N, Noseda A, Jespers P, Melot C, Naeije R, van de Borne P, *Does endothelin play a role in chemoreception during acute hypoxia in normal men?* Chest. 2007 May; 131(5): p.1467-1472.

5. Common CO2 uses for cancer treatment

Is there any experimental or clinical evidence indicating usefulness of CO2 for malignant tumors and cancer? More and more oncologists conduct their clinical investigations with application of CO2-O2 gas mixtures for cancer patients. This mixture is called "carbogen". The mixture usually contains somewhere from 2 to 5% of carbon dioxide and the remaining portion is oxygen (from about 95 to 98%). Carbogen breathing is usually provided for people with cancer for several hours during administration of certain anti-cancer medications. Why would carbogen be useful? The logic is simple: increased CO2 will help to dilate blood vessels (due to CO2 vasodilatory effect) and release more O2 in tumors (due to the enhanced Bohr effect). At the same time, increased O2 will improve oxygenation of the arterial blood due to freely dissolved oxygen (that is toxic in a long run, but can have benefits to save lives).

Let us review some of these results and the claimed reasons for carbogen application. Several studies from England and the USA found that breathing various carbogen mixtures significantly improves oxygenation of tumors. The general opinion of these researchers is presented in the following quote. "*Perfusion insufficiency and the resultant hypoxia are recognized as important mechanisms of resistance to anticancer therapy. Modification of the tumor microenvironment to increase perfusion and oxygenation of tumors may improve on the efficacy of these treatments...*"(Powell et al, 1997).

Obviously, increased perfusion is one of the known CO2 effects due to its vasodilatory powers.

A group of British research scientists from the Paul Strickland Scanner Centre revealed that, when their cancer patients breathed various carbogen mixtures (with 2%, 3.5% and 5% CO2 content, where the remaining part was oxygen), their *"arterial oxygen tension increased at least three-fold from basal values"* (Baddeley et al, 2000). *"There were no significant changes in the respiratory rate, heart rate and blood pH. The results suggest that 2% CO2 in O2 enhances arterial oxygen levels to a similar extent as 3.5% and 5% CO2 and that it is well tolerated"* (Baddeley et al, 2000).

Another group of British researchers directly measured O2 pressure in cancer cells and concluded, *"This study confirms that breathing 2% CO2 and 98% O2 is well tolerated and effective in increasing tumor oxygenation"* (Powell et al, 1999).

These results generate the following question. Which gas is the main contributor to the increased oxygenation of cells, is it O2 or CO2? The content of both gases in used mixtures were much higher than the O2 and CO2 contents in normal air. Therefore, both of them can produce the positive effect on tissue oxygenation.

Let us first consider the possible contribution brought about by the increased oxygen content in inspired air. There are two O2 states in the arterial blood. While breathing normal air, about 98.5 % of all O2 is combined with hemoglobin or red blood cells; and only about 1.5%

of O2 is dissolved in blood plasma (free oxygen). Which among these O2 components is responsible for the main increase in oxygenation of the arterial blood in the carbogen studies?

The saturation of hemoglobin with O2 under normal conditions (or when breathing normal air) is very high or about 98-99 %. Increased O2 pressure can raise this value to almost 100%. This would cause only about a 2% increase in relation to the total normal arterial blood oxygenation. However, the contribution due to freely dissolved O2 can be much greater. In normal conditions the contribution of dissolved O2 is only about 1.5% of the total blood O2. Normal air has about 20% O2. Increasing O2 content in the inspired air (from 20 to 100% or almost five times) can increase freely dissolved oxygen to about 6-7% in relation to the initial value. Hence, increasing the O2 component in the inspired air can cause about 8-9% increase in total O2 content in the arterial blood (with 2% increase for combined oxygen and 6-7% for freely dissolved oxygen).

Could it be so that carbon dioxide is more essential in improving tumor oxygenation? British doctors decided *"to assess the relative contributions of carbon dioxide and oxygen to this response and the tumor oxygenation state, the response of GH3 prolactinomas to 5% CO2/95% air, carbogen and 100% O2"* (Baddeley et al, 2000). That was done using magnetic resonance imaging and PO2 histography or using direct measurements of O2 concentrations. They discovered that, *"A 10-30% image intensity increase was observed during 5% CO2/95% air breathing, consistent with an increase in tumor blood flow, as a result of CO2-induced vasodilation, reducing the concentration of deoxyhemoglobin in the blood. Carbogen caused a further 40-50% signal enhancement, suggesting an additional improvement due to increase blood oxygenation. A small 5-10% increase was observed in response to 100% O2, highlighting the dominance of CO2-induced vasodilation in the carbogen response"* (Baddeley et al, 2000).

They say here that it is not oxygen, but carbon dioxide that is the main substance responsible for the observed improvement in oxygenation of tumors during carbogen breathing. Higher O2 concentrations, while providing additional improvement in oxygenation of the arterial blood and tumors, are toxic for lungs alveoli. It is well known that, due to its high chemical reactivity, oxygen causes oxidative damage to tissues and formation of free radicals. Hence, it is logical to expect that, if the same patients use 100% O2 for many days, not just hours, the oxidative damage can produce more harm for the whole body than the benefits of pure oxygen for tumor reduction. This is the case for people with severe COPD and emphysema who are often prescribed breathing 100% O2 until they die some years later (or learn how to slow down their breathing back to the medical norm.) Higher CO2, on the other hand, can cause sustained improvements in tumor oxygenation without any negative effects.

Indeed, more detailed analysis or dynamic of improved oxygenation was investigated by German scientists from the Institute of Physiology and Pathophysiology at the University of Mainz. In their conclusions, these researchers wrote, *"Higher inspiratory CO2 fractions (2.5 or 5%) lead to a prolonged improvement of tumor perfusion after the end of inspiratory hyperoxia when compared with pure oxygen breathing. Since no principal differences in oxygenation and perfusion were seen between the gases containing 2.5 and 5% CO2, the former may be preferable for inspiratory hyperoxia"* (Thews et al, 2002). They found that positive effects of pure oxygen are very short in duration, while CO2 produces lasting improvement. This is a normal effect due to adaptation of the breathing center to higher arterial CO2.

But a cancer patient can safely increase own arterial CO2 content and oxygenation of the tumors naturally by learning how to breathe less, while preserving normal arterial blood oxygenation (about 98% for O2 hemoglobin saturation) and avoiding oxidative damage, as well as expensive carbogen therapies and time. In addition, since conventional anticancer therapies do not address certain lifestyle factors, their efficiency is low. Why is it so? Most tumors have intensive growth only during certain hours of the day, when the person has their heaviest breathing and lowest body oxygenation. Therefore, the tumor may shrink due to the effect of any anticancer therapy, but it will grow again later.

References

Baddeley H, Brodrick PM, Taylor NJ, Abdelatti MO, Jordan LC, Vasudevan AS, Phillips H, Saunders MI, Hoskin PJ, *Gas exchange parameters in radiotherapy patients during breathing of 2%, 3.5% and 5% carbogen gas mixtures*, Br J Radiol 2000 Oct; 73(874): p. 1100-1104.

Powell ME, Hill SA, Saunders MI, Hoskin PJ, Chaplin DJ, *Human tumour blood flow is enhanced by nicotinamide and carbogen breathing*, Cancer Res 1997 Dec 1; 57(23): p. 5261-5264.

Powell ME, Collingridge DR, Saunders MI, Hoskin PJ, Hill SA, Chaplin DJ, *Improvement in human tumour oxygenation with carbogen of varying carbon dioxide concentrations*, Radiother Oncol 1999 Feb; 50(2): p. 167-171.

Thews O, Kelleher DK, Vaupel P, *Dynamics of tumor oxygenation and red blood cell flux in response to inspiratory hyperoxia combined with different levels of inspiratory hypercapnia*, Radiother Oncol. 2002 Jan; 62(1): p. 77-85.

6. Ukrainian clinical trial: effects of breathing normalization on metastatic breast cancer

6.1 Metastatic cancer is deadly

Metastatic breast cancer is deadly. Complete clinical remission, after application of commonly accepted methods, including surgical removal of tumors and radiation therapy, is rare. In the 1980s, German oncologist Dr. Hartlapp suggested that only 10 to 20% of patients with metastatic breast cancer achieve complete remission (Hartlapp, 1986). During the last decades of the 20th century, there have been changes in survival rates. For example, previously, for studies conducted in the 1970s, it was common to report only about 10% survival at five years for people with metastatic breast cancer. During early 1990s, survival increased up to nearly 30%, and around the year 2000, it was around 40%. Are there any further improvements?

US doctors from the Department of Surgery and Division of Surgical Oncology at the Louisiana State University and the Feist-Weiller Cancer Center in Shreveport, Louisiana measured correlation between one metastatic biomarker chemokine receptor CXCR4 level in a group of 77 women with locally advanced breast cancer. Note that doctors use the term "locally advanced" or "regionally advanced" when they refer to large tumors that usually involve the breast skin and underlying chest structures with changes in the breast's shape, as well as visible or palpable lymph node enlargement. The main danger for this stage of cancer is distant metastasis. Out of 77 patients, "*55 patients (71%) had low CXCR4 level. The 5-year overall survival for the low and high CXCR4 group was 78% and 50%, respectively (P = .015)*" (Hiller et al, 2011). If we combine all participants together, their overall 5-year survival would be about 70%.

We can witness a steady increase in management of cancer even though there is a lot of criticism from general population and people who provide alternative therapies. For example, some alternative health care practitioners may claim that there are no benefits in surgery and radiation therapy even for advanced forms of cancer. However, there are studies that proved usefulness of these commonly accepted anticancer treatment therapies. One such study was done in 2011. Let us review its results.

Since prevention and detection of breast cancer is not advanced in many Asian countries, and many women do not have surgeries even for metastatic breast cancer, a group of Malaysian scientists from the Julius Centre University of Malaya in Kuala Lumpur compared impact of surgery on survival rates. They found, "*The 2-year survival rate was 21.2 per cent in women who did not have surgery and 46.3 per cent in those who had breast surgery*" (Pathy et al, 2011).

This makes total physiological sense since presence of large numbers of malignant cells consume nutrients and other resources from the human organism and produces stress for organs of elimination and the immune system causing increased ventilation, reduced body oxygenation and further advance of cancer.

Since there are different stages for advanced cancer, it is obvious that survival rates are higher for people with early stages of breast cancer, and gets higher for locally advanced and metastatic cancer. For example, if we select a large group of people from a developed country and with earliest stages of metastatic breast cancer, it is normal to expect that their 5-year survival is going to be about 70-80% assuming that they use those techniques suggested by their official healthcare providers.

In addition, cancer is one of the most feared conditions. It produces numerous proven negative effects of workability, sleep, energy levels, and mental and emotional wellbeing of people. The effects of metastatic cancer are even more devastating. However, the Ukrainian breast cancer clinical trial (Paschenko, 2001) dramatically improved survival rates and quality of life in people practicing breathing retraining. Let is review all parts of this monumental clinical investigation.

References

Hiller DJ, Meschonat C, Kim R, Li BD, Chu QD, *Chemokine receptor CXCR4 level in primary tumors independently predicts outcome for patients with locally advanced breast cancer,* Surgery. 2011 Sep;150(3):459-65.

Paschenko S, *Study of application of the reduced breathing method in a combined treatment of breast cancer,* Oncology (Kiev, Ukraine) 2001, v. 3, No.1, p. 77-78.

Pathy NB, Verkooijen HM, Taib NA, Hartman M, Yip CH, *Impact of breast surgery on survival in women presenting with metastatic breast cancer,* Br J Surg. 2011 Nov;98(11):1566-72.

6.2 Background and introduction

This clinical trial was conducted by Dr. Sergey Paschenko, MD, a pupil of Dr. Konstantin Buteyko (the author of the Buteyko breathing method). Dr. Paschenko was a participant of the 2nd Buteyko Conference organized for medical professionals practicing the Buteyko breathing self-oxygenation therapy.

His study on cancer was published by the Ukrainian National Journal of Oncology (Kiev), and its title was "Study of application of the reduced breathing method in a combined treatment of breast cancer" (Paschenko, 2001). Before going into the details of this study, let us review its introduction since it helps us to understand Dr Paschenko views on causes of cancer and reasons behind application of breathing retraining.

Dr. Paschenko started his article with review of medical literature claiming that low O2 stimulates growth of tumors. He stated that hyperventilation is developed during proliferation of malignant tumors. In my view, tissue hypoxia and hyperventilation exist even before first groups of malignant cells evolve, while it is absolutely correct that presence of pathological masses of cells further worsen breathing. Dr. Paschenko described hypocapnia as the key factor in advancing cancer. He mentioned a shift of the curve of blood hemoglobin dissociation due to low CO2 implying the Bohr effect discussed above. However, he did not mention the vasoconstrictive effects of hypocapnia that can be the leading factor causing tissue hypoxia in body cells and tumors.

It is hard to predict, without detailed clinical investigations, the exact contributions of these two effects (vasodialtion vs. the Bohr effect) on cancer tumors. Oxygen transport is essentially controlled by vasodilation-vasoconstriction effect (that regulates perfusion of organs and tissues) and the Bohr effect (that regulates oxygen release in capillaries). Even in normal tissues, the presence of other factors, such as the relaxation of smooth muscles of blood vessels and the metabolic activity in tissues, influence both blood flow and affinity of red blood cells to hemoglobin. In tumors, this picture is much more complex due to variety of causes including large pH changes caused by activities of malignant cells.

Then Dr. Paschenko stated that "*normal breathing improves quality of life in patients with malignant tumors and increases the efficiency of special anticancer treatment*". Therefore, he suggested to use those methods that slow down breathing and leads to increased CO_2 and O_2 concentrations in body cells. Dr. Paschenko mentioned therapeutical values of yoga and autogenic training due to relaxation of muscles and gradual breathing normalization. Another crucial factor that was mentioned by him in introduction was physical exercise that increases oxygenation of tumors, metabolism and cellular immunity.

6.3 Subjects and methods of the trial

In this study, Dr. Paschenko applied reduced breathing exercises in order to recondition the breathing center to breathing less air and increase CO_2 content in the lungs and body cells. Reduced breathing sessions are based on breathing slightly less than usual, while having correct posture and an empty stomach. Instead of having large inhalations, the patient is suggested to have shorter inhalations using only the diaphragm and exhalations accompanied by relaxation. This reduced breathing results in a light, but comfortable desire to breathe more (or air hunger) coupled with relaxation of the diaphragm for exhalations. All other parts and muscles of the human body should be also relaxed in order to facilitate adaptation of the breathing center to higher CO_2. In this clinical trial, the total duration of breathing exercises ranged from 60 minutes up to 2.5-4 hours per day for 3 years.

Single breathing sessions ranged from 20 to 30 min in duration. However, it is known to all Buteyko practitioners that just practicing breathing exercises does not guarantee steady improvements in breathing parameters of learners. Addressing lifestyle risk factors is a very important part of breathing normalization. Furthermore, for many groups of people, lifestyle changes (related to, for example, sleep, exercise, and diet) are necessary for permanent normalization of automatic breathing. In addition, there are focal infections that can prevent any progress in breathing normalization and better body oxygenation. All these changes are parts of the Buteyko reduced breathing technique.

Even though these methods are not mentioned in this study, I have no doubts that Dr. Paschenko used numerous supplementary methods required for breathing retraining. One hundred twenty patients with breast cancer (T1-2N1M0) participated in this trial. These letters and numbers relate to international classification of stages of breast cancer. T1-2 means that the tumors are less than 5 cm or 2 inches in size. N1 means that cancer has spread to 1 to 3 axillary (underarm) lymph nodes and/or tiny amounts of cancer are found in internal mammary lymph nodes (those near the breast bone) on sentinel lymph node biopsy. M0 signifies no distant metastasis. All patients had a standard anticancer therapy that included surgical removal of tumors. However, in addition to this therapy, the breathing retraining group (67 patients) practiced breathing exercises (together with lifestyle changes, as discussed above). Their parameters were compared with the control group (the remaining 53 patients) at the base level and after 1, 2 and 3 years.

6.4 Results and discussion

All people with cancer suffer from tissue hypoxia caused, as numerous studies indicate, by their heavy and fast automatic breathing. This causes low CO_2 concentrations in the alveoli of the lungs, arterial blood and expired air. As we discussed above, before the treatment, the average amount of CO_2 in the expired air for all patients was about 2.9±0.3% ($p>0.05$) indicating severe hyperventilation. The approximate numbers for minute ventilation would be over 15 liters per minute instead of 6.

Changes in expired CO_2 concentrations during this 3-year trial are presented in this table.

Time period	Control group	Breathing group
Initial	2.7±0.2%	3.1±0.3%
Surgery + chemotherapy	2.4±0.2%	2.5±0.3%
1 year follow-up	3.1±0.3%	4.3±0.5%
2 years follow-up	3.1±0.3%	5.1+0.5%
3 years follow-up	3.1±0.3%	5.5±0.6%

CO2 content during the cancer trial

As Dr. Paschenko noted, standard medical treatment that included chemotherapy resulted in slight further fall in

CO2 content. It is known that chemotherapy produces a powerful shock that may take weeks to recover. We can assume here that even heavier and faster breathing is the expected effect of chemotherapy. Nearly all common prolonged adverse symptoms experienced after chemotherapy can be quickly eliminated using breathing retraining. Therefore, it is well known among Buteyko breathing practitioners that breathing retraining helps to have quick health recovery immediately after chemotherapy.

During the following 3 years, as the table shows, the breathing retraining program resulted in a steady increase in expired CO2 content in the control group. After 3 years of breathing normalization, the control group even exceeded the official medical norm for end-tidal (and arterial CO2) of 5.3%. Therefore, the results show that they started to breathe less air than the clinical norm.

However, Dr. Paschenko observed that there were participants who could not increase their CO2 above 5%. This related to patients who were 50 years or older. Very slow CO2 increase was observed in those participants who had additional pathologies, such as hypertension, stenocardia, or diabetes mellitus. (In fact, I believe that these were the only participants who did not survive.) Another practical observation relates to those participants who had metastasis to distant tissues during this trial. In such cases, their CO2 content fell down to 1.5-2% indicating severe uncontrollable hyperventilation.

Apart from higher CO2 concentrations, the breathing retraining group improved their quality of life that included disappearance of fear of unfavorable outcomes of the treatment, improved working ability, and easier social adaptation. There were 9 participants in each group with edema of their upper extremities. Elimination of deep breathing led to disappearance of edema. Dr. Paschenko also reported, "*As the CO2 concentration in the expired air increased from to 4.5-5%, we observed an increased resistance of the organism: reduced inflammatory and allergic processes in the upper respiratory airways, reduced blood pressure, less frequent chest pain, and improved working ability and physical endurance*". Finally, three-year survival rate after application of the combined treatment (surgeries, chemotherapy and breathing normalization) was 95.5% in patients of the main group, and 75.5% in the control group ($p<0.05$). I doubt that there are currently any known metastatic cancer trials that had the same success. There were only 3 participants of this trial who died during these 3 years. According to the description of the article, it is very likely that these people had serous accompanying health problems such as heart disease and diabetes.

From the experience of Russian and Soviet Buteyko medical doctors, as well as my own experience with my students, people with combined or complex conditions are the most difficult category of students since many of them cannot slow down their breathing due to too much stress imposed by diseases. The results for their body oxygen test remain the same even after practicing best breathing exercises that they can perform for up to 30-40 minutes. Therefore, should Dr. Paschenko have a stricter criteria for the participants of this trial (without people with serious additional pathologies), he could have gotten 100%

survival rate. This would mean that self-oxygenation therapies based on breathing normalization are the most influential among currently availabel supplementary anticancer techniques.

6.5 The Buteyko method: chief self-oxygenation therapy

The Buteyko method is the most advanced medical self-oxygenation therapy due to two main reasons:

1. It applies the body oxygen test or control pause to measure effects of breathing exercises and lifestyle changes. Therefore, each person can easily monitor his or her daily, weekly and monthly progress in breathing retraining.

2. It applies a variety of effective and highly developed techniques to address virtually all lifestyle parameters that relate to sleep, diet, exercise, posture, thermoregulation, and many other things that are crucial for easy breathing and increased body oxygenation 24/7.

Dr. Buteyko trained about 200 medical professionals to apply the Buteyko method. In 1985, the Ministry of Health approved the Buteyko breathing technique for the treatment of bronchial asthma. According to official statistic of the Buteyko Clinic in Moscow, the technique has been applied by medical doctors or MDs on more than 100,000 asthmatics, over 30,000 people with cardiovascular problems and thousands of patients with other conditions (bronchitis, diabetes, cancer, HIV, liver cirrhosis, etc.).

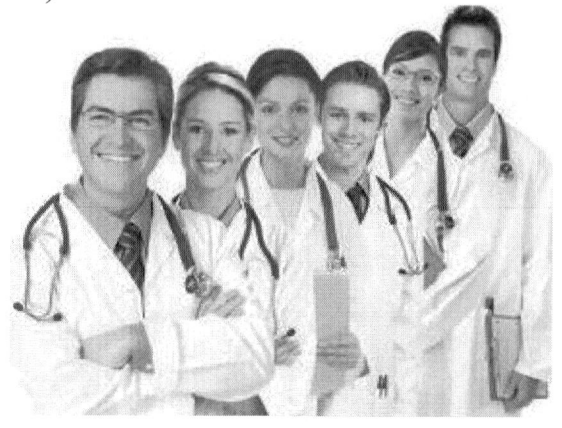

The Buteyko breathing technique has had several successful clinical trials on asthma (England, Australia, New Zealand, Canada, Ukraine, USSR) with average reduction in medication of about 70-90%. Bear in mind that an average participant of these trials even did not achieve the official medical norm for breathing. After 3-6 months of practice, they could get only about half way towards the norm.

In addition to these Western trials, there were several Soviet medical approbations and trials of the Buteyko method, Here is their list:

• 1981, Sechenov's Med Inst, Moscow, USSR (asthma with pneumonia, rhinitis, chronic tonsillitis)

- 1990, Shevchenko's Central Hospital, Kiev, Ukraine (radiation disease)

- 1991, Kiev Scientific and Research Institute of Epidemiology and Infectious Diseases, Ukraine (HIV-AIDS)

- 1991, Kiev Scient and Res Inst of Epidemiol and Infect Diseases, Ukraine (hepatitis B and liver cirrhosis)
- 2001 Zaporozhsky State Institute of Further Medical Education, Zaporozhie, Ukraine (cancer - discussed above).

The organizers of these clinical trials reported significant improvements in health state and symptoms or even complete clinical remission in participants who managed to achieve normal breathing. This is also true for people with cancer. Since there were dozens of medical doctors trained by Dr. K. Buteyko to teach his method to their patients, clearly, there were hundreds of Soviet and Russian patients who had cancer and used this technique as a supplementary therapy.

The general observations of these doctors are following. Breathing normalization is able to prevent and even eliminate existing single tumors and even early stages of metastatic cancer. However, when malignant cells are present in distant tissues (stages 3 and 4), the Buteyko method and breathing exercises allow more peaceful death and much better state of mind during last days and weeks of life. There are possibly people who can survive and defeat cancer even though they have minimum invasion to distant tissues, while using conventional medical methods and breathing techniques. However, new studies and more work are required to find the exact border (for different types of cancer) that separates those who can survive and live and those whose chances of survival are miniscule.

7. Other self-oxygenation therapies

7.1 Frolov breathing device

When people use the Buteyko breathing method, they measure their progress using the body oxygen test that is also called the CP (control pause). Dr. Buteyko, when he conducted his respiratory studies and invented the Buteyko method, did not use the CP test. His had devices to measure exhaled CO_2 as well as many other respiratory parameters in his subjects. As Dr. Buteyko correctly observed, that it is not important what you do, it is more important where you arrive as a result of your breathing exercises.

Vladimir Fedorovich Frolov knew about the discoveries of Dr. Buteyko and the beneficial effects of CO_2 on the human body. Vladimir Frolov graduated from the Military Academy of Chemical Defense in Moscow and worked in the area of development and production of devices for chemical defense. Well educated in the areas of biochemistry and medicine, Vladimir Frolov was an author of 6 patented practical inventions.

In late 1980's, he got an "idea about creation of the Device for Each Person". In his book "Endogenous breathing: medicine of the third millennium", he wrote, "... the Buteyko method could become the scientific foundation for such device. According to Buteyko, diseases appear due to carbon dioxide deficiency in the arterial blood". This is how and why the idea of creation the Frolov breathing device was born. It was invented by Vladimir

Fedorovich Frolov and Eugene Fedorovich Kustov in the 1990's. Numerous Russian clinical trials and approbations have found that the Frolov device is safe and effective medical tool to reduce symptoms and medication for various health problems (including asthma, bronchitis, COPD, emphysema, hypertension, angina pectoris, sinusitis, diabetes, arthritis, seizures, sleep apnea, and other conditions). In Russia, the Frolov breathing device can be bought in pharmacies and hundreds of Russian MDs or family physicians prescribe the Frolov breathing device to their patients so that they can buy and use it.

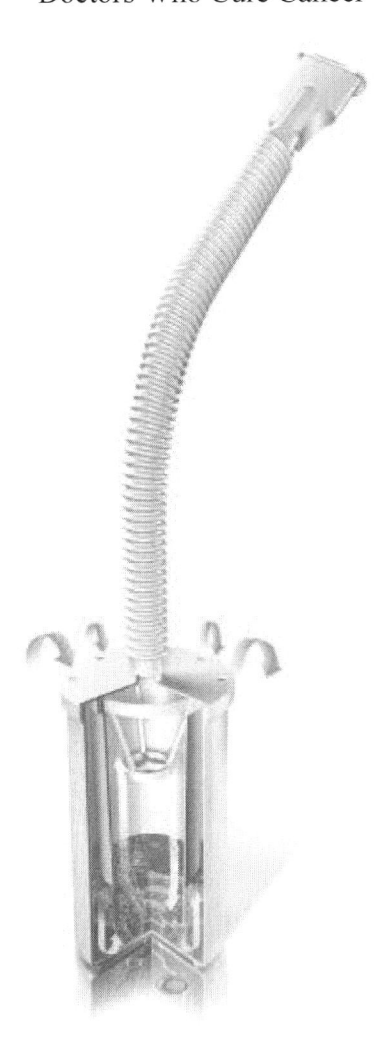

There were no clinical trials on cancer with the Frolov device yet, but over 300 health professionals (MDs, GPs or family physicians, nurses, physiotherapists, and other medical professionals) have been involved in studying, endorsement and promotion of the Frolov breathing device and its application to their patients in Russia since year 2000.

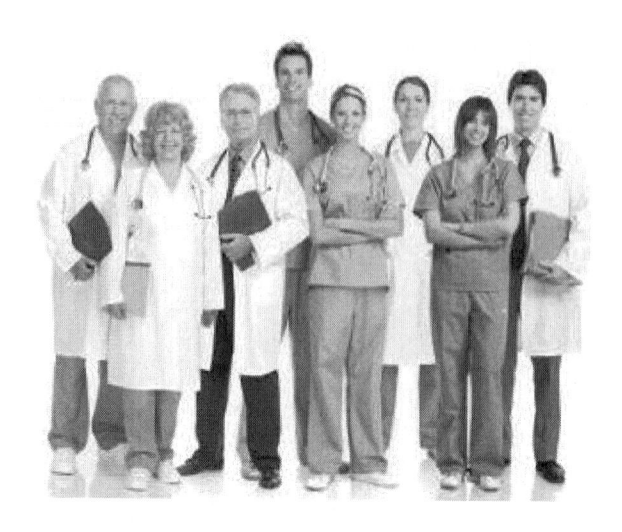

According to the largest world's producer of the Frolov breathing devices company Dinamika http://www.intellectbreathing.com/, more than 2,000,000 people in Russia could confirm that they have improved their health with the help of the Frolov Respiration Training Device, implying the goals set have been successfully achieved.

Apart from two patents in the USSR and Russia, the Frolov respiration device was patented in the USA - Patent Number 5,755,640 (here is a PDF file: 1998 USA Frolov Device Patent). In the USA, since 2000 the Frolov breathing device was officially approved by the US FDA (Food and Drug Administration) as a Class 2 medical device (Frolov FDA's approval).

There are two following advantages of the Frolov device in comparison with Buteyko breathing exercises:

1. For nearly all people with heavy breathing and low body O2 content, cancer patients included, the Frolov device about 1.5-2 times more effective meaning that you need to spend much less time, while being able to achieve the same final results

2. There is no need to have a breathing teacher or practitioner in order to practice breathwork with the Frolov device.

7.2 How Does the Frolov Breathing Device Work?

The main principle is relatively simple: when we breathe in and out through the device, we get a different air composition in our lungs. In normal conditions, when we breathe usual air, the air that we inhale has about 21% of oxygen and 0.03% of carbon dioxide. If we start to breathe through any device, in and out, the device traps a portion of the exhaled air. This exhaled air has less O2 and more CO2. For example, if we collect all exhaled air of the ordinary healthy man during normal breathing, it will contain about 15.3% O2 and 4.2% CO2 since the human body uses O2 and generates CO2 24/7.

When we breathe only through the device (inhalations and exhalations), there are changes in the air composition that enters our lungs depending on the parameters of our breathing and device. Indeed, during our exhalation, part of the exhaled air is trapped in the breathing device. Furthermore, the initial part of the exhaled gas has almost no extra CO2 and about 21% O2 since this air does not participate in gas exchange. (Ironically, it is called "dead volume", but in reality it is a factor promoting health due to drastic changes in air compositions during Earth's evolution). The last portion of the exhaled air has highest CO2 content and lowest O2 values. Hence, the device can trap this last portion of the exhaled air, which has high CO2 concentration (up to about 5-6% in healthy people) and much less oxygen (about 14-15%) than in normal air. Hence, during our next inhalation, when we breathe only through the device, this trapped air mixes with fresh air.

Hence, most people can more safely practice deep breathing (e.g., by having 3-5 large deep breaths in one minute) when using the device without problems with low CO2 in the lungs and other body cells. The approximate composition of the inhaled air during breathing sessions is provided in this Table:

Inhaled air composition before and during breathing sessions

Gas in air	Inhaled normal air	Inhaled air during breathing sessions
CO2 content	0.03% CO2	1-2% CO2
O2 content	20% O2	18-19% O2

The exact composition of the inhaled air is difficult to predict because it depends on many parameters:

1) volume of trapped air in the plastic bottle (the larger this volume, the higher the inhaled CO_2 and the lower the exhaled O_2);

2) amplitude of breathing (it is called tidal volume);

3) breathing frequency (it is considered in the next section);

4) metabolic rate (or CO_2-generation rate).

Those people, who inhale through the nose and exhale through the device, do not use air that is trapped in the device for their breathing. However, since they try to make longer exhalations, their lungs naturally accumulate more CO_2 and have less O_2. Hence, they experience a similar physiological effect, but to a smaller degree.

Therefore, Frolov device breathing exercise is a type of **intermittent hypercapnic hypoxic training**:

"intermittent" means that it is done only for about 15-20 minutes, but the effects are lasting for many following hours; "hypercapnic" indicates higher CO_2 levels in the alveoli of the lungs during sessions (CO_2 concentration in the arterial blood and body cells also gets higher if there is no ventilation-perfusion mismatch); and "hypoxic" implies temporary reduced oxygen content in the alveoli.

Similar effects (more CO2 and less O2 in the inhaled air) take place during other beneficial forms of breathing exercises: Buteyko breathing exercises and Pranayama (a slow deep breathing exercise from hatha yoga). However, the breathing device has some advantages: it allows active movements of the respiratory muscles (mainly the diaphragm) and, as a result, it is much easier to tolerate higher CO2 and lower O2 concentrations in the lungs and blood. Active muscular diaphragmatic movements, together with variations in internal pressure during inhalations and exhalations, gently stimulate all internal organs and lymph nodes located under the diaphragm as during intensive physical exercise. Furthermore, the device causes gentle or gradual CO2 increase, while Pranayama breath holds and Buteyko breath holds lead to sudden CO2 upsurge, which can cause problems to some groups of people. Hypoxic training (less O2 in the inhaled air) without hypercapnia takes place when athletes and other people breathe air and live at high altitude (1,500-3,000 m above the sea level).

A short breathing session (e.g., 3-5 minutes) with the Frolov breathing device leads to quick reduction in acute symptoms of many chronic diseases (including exacerbation of asthma, bronchitis, headache, chest pain due to angina, blocked nose, chronic coughing, pain due to arthritis, dyspnea, constipation, shortness of breath, and seizures).

People with cancer report immediate and lasting reduction in dyspnea and increased feeling of energy. Typical breathing sessions (15 min or longer) produce a profound and lasting rejuvenating effect due to boosted body oxygenation with improved focus, sleep, digestion and many other physiological and biochemical parameters. Systematic applications of the Frolov breathing device, combined with healthy lifestyle changes, leads to steady increase in CO2 and gradual restoration of normal breathing. As soon as someone achieves the same CO2 concentrations as for the Ukrainian clinical trial on cancer, this person can expect the same results related to survival and quality of life.

If you decide to use the Frolov device, keep in mind that it is smart to apply those lifestyle changes that are endorsed by the Buteyko method and use the body oxygen test that provides you with vital real-time information about your overall progress.

7.3 Amazing DIY breathing device

It is possible to regulate the amount of water in the Frolov breathing device for breathing exercises. Therefore, this device has adjustable resistance for exhalations. (The effects of water volumes on inhalation resistance is small.) Each person with cancer has a certain initial respiratory characteristics. And the purpose of breathing normalization is to improve these characteristics towards the medical norms. However, as with any type of long-term learning and training, we need to apply mild but persistent efforts. In order to be effective, the training process should present us with a mild but accomplishable stress of resistance so that we get better.

The Frolov device covers a wide range of such initial parameters due to an ability to use variable amounts of water in its inner container. (The amount of water in the Frolov device regulates its resistance during exhalations.) Therefore, it is a perfectly suitable device for up to 80-90% of people with cancer and other disorders. There are however severely sick people (many people with metastatic cancer, people with serious respiratory problems such as advanced COPD and emphysema, people after heart attack and stroke, and some others) who can find that it is too difficult to use the Frolov device even with the minimum amount of water. These groups of people can use the modified Frolov breathing technique with inhalations through the nose and slow exhalations through the device.

Another option for such severely sick and weak people is to make a DIY breathing device that I have been using for hundreds of my students for about 2 years. I call it the Amazing DIY breathing device due to its power to boost body oxygenation. Here is a picture of the Amazing DIY breathing device.

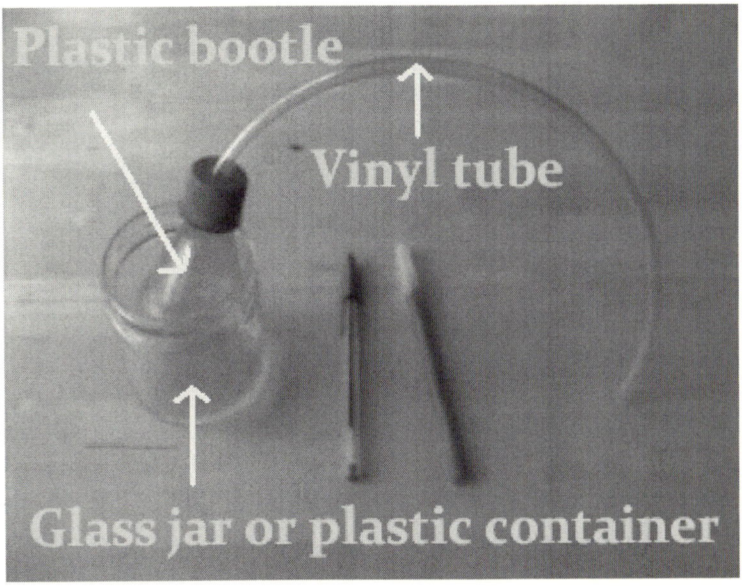
Plastic bootle
Vinyl tube
Glass jar or plastic container

The key advantage of the Amazing DIY breathing device is in its ability to regulate its resistance by using different diameters and length of vinyl tubing that can be easily bought in hardware and gardening stores.

The DIY device can be made easier than the Frolov device with minimum amount of water, or the DIY device can be made harder (or more resistive) than the Frolov device with maximum amount of water (30 ml).

Obviously, one needs to know how to make the right device, and this process is explained in details in the book "Amazing DIY Breathing Device" - http://www.normalbreathing.com/book-DIY-breathing-device.php.

7.4 Can yoga be used for self-oxygenation?

Correctly done yoga is another excellent tool to boost body oxygenation and fight cancer. The main problem is that leading modern yoga teachers distorted and perverted the essence of traditional ancient yoga. First of all, it is taught or implied now that yoga postures or asanas are more important than breathing. Second, when thinking about breathing, yoga teachers and yoga students think about breathing exercises instead of correct breathing 24/7. It is not important how you breathe during 1 or even 2-3 hours of breathing exercises. It is much more important how you breathe during remaining 20+ hours of the day, and especially how you breathe during night sleep. Finally, most yoga teachers promote the deep breathing myth saying and assuming that breathing more air is good for better body oxygenation and health, while CO_2 is toxic gas that we need to expel from the body cells and lungs. Meanwhile, traditional yoga has always been about breathing slower and less. Here are some quotes from ancient yoga textbooks that are also called Sanscrit manuscripts.

Hatha Yoga Pradipika (15 century)

"3. So long as the (breathing) air stays in the body, it is called life. Death consists in passing out of the (breathing) air. It is, therefore, necessary to restrain the breath."
"17. Hiccough, asthma, cough, pain in the head, the ears, and the eyes; these and other various kinds of diseases are generated by the disturbance of the breath."
"28. The breathing is calmed when the mind becomes steady and calm; ..."

The Gheranda Samhita (15-17 century)

"7. Wherever the yogi may be, he should always, in everything he does, be sure to keep the tongue upwards and constantly hold the breath. This is Nabhomudra, the destroyer of diseases for yogis."

The Yoga Sutra of Patanjali (4th-2nd century BC)

"Pranayama [the main breathing exercise in yoga] is the cessation of inspiratory and expiratory movements."
There are no any suggestions in these main classical yoga texts about breathing more air and expelling some poisons from the lungs. The most important yoga breathing exercise pranayama is done with maximum breath holds before and after inhalations. There are other versions of pranayama, but they all have the same general idea: the yoga student needs to breathe less air than before the practice. another crucial requirement in pranayama is gradual elongation of all phases of breathing.

The Shiva Samhita (17-18 century)

(5) The Pranayama

"22. Then let the wise practitioner close with his right thumb the pingala (right nostril), inspire air through the ida (the left nostril); and keep the air confined – suspend his breathing – as long as he can; and afterwards let him breathe out slowly, and not forcibly, through the right nostril."

Increase of Duration

"53. Then gradually he should make himself able to practice for three gharis (one hour and a half at a time, he should be able to restrain breath for that period). Through this, the Yogi undoubtedly obtains all the longed for powers."

"57. When he gets the power of holding breath (i.e., to be in a trance) for three hours, then certainly the wonderful state of pratyahar is reached without fail."

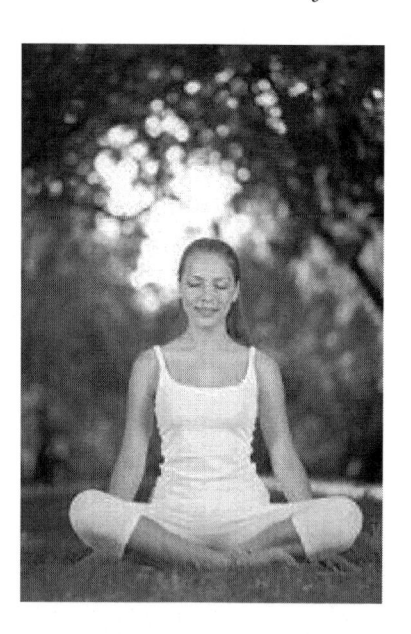

Now we can certainly explain what is going on with automatic breathing of yoga students. During each breathing session, due to breath holds and slower breathing, they accumulate more CO_2 in the lungs and body cells. This causes slower and lighter breathing after breathing sessions and increased body O2 content. Furthermore, when they practice yoga breathing exercises for weeks and months, they gradually reset their breathing center to higher CO2 concentrations. This means that their basal breathing becomes slower and lighter, while body oxygenation gets higher and higher.

In addition to breathwork, most asanas were selected by ancient yoga teachers with the same final result: to achieve slower and lighter breathing. If you practice yoga and pay attention to the way you breathe, you can easily discover that nearly all asanas make you to hold your breath naturally. This is the reason why yoga novices can do most asanas, like bridge, cobra, and others only while they hold their breath or only for some 7-10 seconds. Later, when they persist with this very wise healing practice, they have slower breathing at rest, more O2 in tissues and can practice the same asanas for longer periods of time.

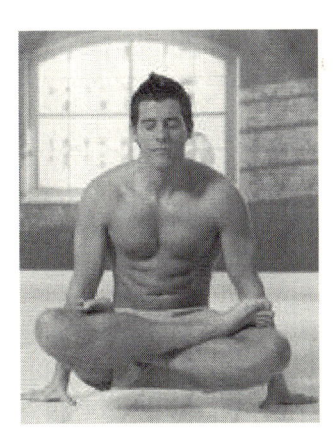

Therefore, if the yoga student knows what to do with his or her breathing during any yoga practice (including hatha yoga, hot yoga, and many others) then they have higher and higher CO2 concentrations in exhaled air and more O2 in cells of the body. This is exactly the key factor to deal with cancer and gain normal or even ideal health.

7.5 Earthing: free electrons increase body O2 and fight tumors

Earthing (electrical grounding of the human body) is an additional positive factor to increase body O2 and fight cancer. It provides free electrons for the human body that act like antioxidants to suppress inflammation, reduce pain and stress, and normalize nerve, muscle, and immune function. Many my students found this technique beneficial. For novices (ungrounded people), just sitting and standing barefoot for 30 min can increase body O2 by 2-5 seconds. Even better results are common for people grounded during sleep. In a long run, an average student can get up to 5-10 s higher morning CPs (body O2) due to correct application of Earthing.

Earthing is a totally natural and powerful supplementary method that was endorsed by Dr. Buteyko and his colleagues. However, they suggested that main benefits of barefoot activities are due to stimulation of nerve endings on soles of feet.

Earthing is not a substitute for other lifestyle factors. Therefore, we still require exercise with nose breathing, correct posture, prevention of supine sleep, clean air, good thermoregulation, an empty stomach (for nearly all people) before going to bed, and many other factors in order to have high body O2 test results for the next morning.

How does grounding work? The electrically insulated human body has a tendency to accumulate positive electrical charge (up to many 100s or 1,000 Volts), while Earth has a slightly negative charge (or excess of electrons). Many antioxidants, like vitamin C, vitamin E, lutein and others, are able to disactivate free radicals (reactive oxygen species) by using only one mechanism: donation to free radicals their free electrons. Electrons provided by Earth produce a similar effect on free radicals as these antioxidants. Therefore, Earthing is a very important additional method to fight cancer and increase body oxygenation.

When the human body has physical contact or electrically connected with Earth, Earth provides unlimited source of free electrons to quench any inflammation and normalize the work of the nervous system and muscles. Preliminary results indicate that Earthing has direct effects on reduction of tumors.

There are several causes that lead to accumulation of a large positive charge (especially due to wearing synthetic clothes) on a human body:

- insulation of the human body (due to wearing modern insulated shoes, walking on wooden and carpet floors, sleeping on elevated beds)

- triboelectricity (especially due to wearing synthetic clothes and walking on carpets)

- induced body currents due to large outer electric and magnetic fields caused by ordinary electric cables, working home appliances, cell phones, laptops, iPads, iPods, and many others.

Depending on their presence and magnitude, these factors lead to electron deficiency that fuels chronic inflammation, pain, abnormalities in transmission of electrical signals in the nervous system and muscles, and other pathological effects. For more details related to Earthing and how to ground yourself (for nearly free using simple DIY methods) – visit this web page: Earthing - http://www.normalbreathing.com/e/earthing.php.

8. Conclusions

Available medical evidence that include hundreds of studies indicate cancer is controlled by body O2 levels. People with cancer have ineffective breathing patterns based on chronic overbreathing. Breathing too much air causes low CO2 values in the lungs, arterial blood and other body cells.

Hypocapnia or reduced CO2 levels produce numerous adverse effects including constriction of blood vessels and reduced release of oxygen in cells due to the suppressed Bohr effect. Therefore, low body oxygenation in people with cancer is the direct result of their heavy breathing at rest. Tissue hypoxia promote growth of tumors and their metastasis. Additionally, low O2 in cells reduces efficiency of other therapies that are used to treat cancer.

Addressing problems related to heavy and deep breathing at rest should be the central part of any anticancer therapy. Breathing normalization methods include breathing exercises and lifestyle changes that make breathing slower and easier, and body O2 values higher.

There are different breathing exercises and methods that can increase O2 levels in tumors and body cells within 10-20 minutes. The purpose of these breathing exercises, together with lifestyle changes, is to achieve permanent changes in automatic breathing patterns. That causes higher CO2 and O2 levels in tissues. This gradual process is the foundation of breathing normalization.

Among the techniques that result in easier breathing are the Buteyko breathing exercises, Frolov breathing device, Amazing DIY breathing device, Oxygen Remedy, hatha yoga pranayama, and some others. Note that the most important part is where you are going to arrive as a result of your activities. This process of breathing normalization often takes many months or even years in people with serious health problems such as cancer. In addition, there are many hidden factors that can slow down breathing retaining such as cortisol deficiency, lack of vital nutrients, lifestyle risk factors (mouth breathing, chest breathing, supine sleep, and so forth), focal infections (including cavities in teeth, root canals, and some other specific problems). All these factors are to be addressed using known methods and techniques from the Buteyko breathing therapy.

More detailed information about most effective breathing exercises, correct lifestyle modifications and other necessary changes in order to achieve normal breathing and defeat cancer using body O2 are provided in Part 2 of this series "Anticancer Program: Boost Body O2 Naturally" (in preparation - April 2012).

About the author: Dr. Artour Rakhimov

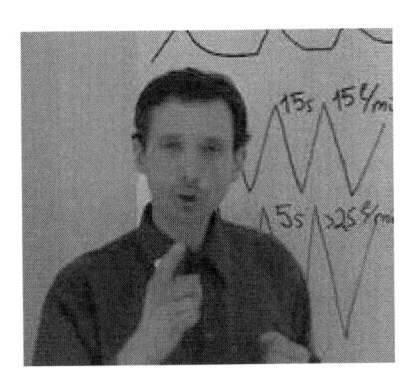

* High School Honor student (Grade "A" for all exams)
* Moscow University Honor student (Grade "A" for all exams)
* Moscow University PhD (Math/Physics), accepted in Canada and the UK
* Winner of many regional competitions in mathematics, chess and sport orienteering (during teenage and University years)
* Good classical piano-player: Chopin, Bach, Tchaikovsky, Beethoven, Strauss (up to now)
* Former captain of the ski-O varsity team and member of the cross-country skiing varsity team of the Moscow State University, best student teams of the USSR
* Former individual coach of world-elite athletes from Soviet (Russian) and Finnish national teams who took gold and silver medals during World Championships
* Total distance covered by running, cross country skiing, and swimming: over 100,000 km or over 2.5 loops around the Earth
* Joined Religious Society of Friends (Quakers) in 2001
* Author of the publication which won Russian National 1998 Contest of scientific and methodological sport papers
* Author of the books, as well as an author of the bestselling Amazon books:
  - "Oxygenate Yourself: Breathe Less" (Buteyko Books; 94 pages; ISBN: 0954599683; 2008; Hardcover)

Dr. Artour Rakhimov

- "Cystic Fibrosis Life Expectancy: 30, 50, 70, ..." *2012 - Amazon Kindle book*
- "Doctors Who Cure Cancer" *2012 - Amazon Kindle book*
- "Yoga Benefits Are in Breathing Less" *2012 - Amazon Kindle book*
- "Crohn's Disease and Colitis: Hidden Triggers and Symptoms" *2012 - Amazon Kindle book*
- "How to Use Frolov Breathing Device (Instructions)" *- 2012 - PDF and Amazon book (120 pages)*
- "Amazing DIY Breathing Device" *- 2010-2012 - PDF and Amazon book*
- "What Science and Professor Buteyko Teach Us About Breathing" *2002*
- "Breathing, Health and Quality of Life" *2004 (91 pages; Translated in Danish and Finnish)*
- "Doctor Buteyko Lecture at the Moscow State University" *2009 (55 pages; Translation from Russian with Dr. A. Rakhimov's comments)*
- "Normal Breathing: the Key to Vital Health" *2009 (The most comprehensive world's book on Buteyko breathing retraining method; over 190,000 words; 305 pages)*

* Author of the world's largest website devoted to breathing, breathing techniques, and breathing retraining (www.NormalBreathing.com)
* Author of numerous YouTube videos (http://www.youtube.com/user/artour2006)
* Buteyko breathing teacher (since 2002 up to now) and trainer
* Inventor of the Amazing DIY breathing device and numerous contributions to breathing retraining
* Whistleblower and investigator of mysterious murder-suicides, massacres and other crimes organized worldwide by GULAG KGB agents using the fast total mind control method
* Practitioner of the New Decision Therapy and Kantillation
* Level 2 Trainer of the New Decision Therapy
* Health writer and health educator

Made in the USA
San Bernardino, CA
02 February 2015